# Estrogen and Breast Cancer

# Estrogen and Breast Cancer

## A Warning to Women

## Carol Ann Rinzler

Foreword by Graham A. Colditz, M.D.

MACMILLAN PUBLISHING COMPANY
NEW YORK
MAXWELL MACMILLAN CANADA
TORONTO
MAXWELL MACMILLAN INTERNATIONAL
NEW YORK   OXFORD   SINGAPORE   SYDNEY

Macmillan Publishing Company     Maxwell Macmillan Canada, Inc.
866 Third Avenue                 1200 Eglinton Avenue East
New York, NY 10022               Suite 200
                                 Don Mills, Ontario M3C 3N1

Macmillan Publishing Company is part of the Maxwell Communication Group of Companies.

Library of Congress Cataloging-in-Publication Data
Rinzler, Carol Ann.
    Estrogen and breast cancer: a warning to women / Carol Ann
    Rinzler.
        p.    cm.
    Includes bibliographical references and index.
    ISBN 0-02-603491-3
    1. Breast—Cancer—Etiology.   2. Breast—Cancer—Prevention.
3. Estrogen—Therapeutic use—Side effects.   4. Oral
contraceptives—Side effects.   I. Title.
    RC280.B8R566       1993              92-43809       CIP
    616.99′449071—dc20

Macmillan books are available at special discounts for bulk purchases for sales promotions, premiums, fund-raising, or educational use. For details, contact:

                    Special Sales Director
                    Macmillan Publishing Company
                    866 Third Avenue
                    New York, NY 10022

10 9 8 7 6 5 4 3 2

Printed in the United States of America

## A Note to the Reader

*For my father,*
*Harold Jerome Rinzler,*
*and my husband,*
*Perry Luntz,*
*who, each in his own way,*
*always encouraged me*
*to say what I know to be right.*

# Contents

Foreword by Graham A. Colditz, M.D.                    xi

Acknowledgments                                        xv

Introduction                                           xvii


## I   Estrogen

1. The Female Principle                                 3
2. Medicine for Menopause, 1930–1960                   13
3. Reproductive Remedies, 1937–1960                    21
4. Problems with The Pill, 1961–1962                   35
5. Menopause Revisited, 1963–1966                      45
6. An Inference of Blame, 1966–1969                    51


## II   Definitions, Statistics, and Studies

7. Defining the Disease                                57
8. Counting the Cases                                  61

## III   Hormones and Cancer

9. The Trail of Evidence, 1961–1969                71
10. Marking Time, 1969–1971                        79
11. First Reckoning, 1975                          89

## IV   The Pill and Breast Cancer

12. An Important Warning, 1970–1975               101
13. The Official Truth, 1980–1987                 113
14. Real Risk, Real Victims, 1986–1991            119

## V   ERT and Breast Cancer

15. No Protection, 1976–1981                      137
16. Confirming Evidence, 1989–1991                151
17. Defending ERT, 1980–1991                      159
18. The Fatal Connection, 1992                    167

## VI   An Agenda for Women

19. Women's Rights, Women's Lives                 173

*Appendix A. Estrogens and Breast Cancer: A Chronology*   191
*Appendix B. Estrogens and Cancer: Studies That Show*
   *the Connection*                               197
*Notes*                                           201
*Bibliography*                                    219
*Index*                                           225

# Foreword

The rapidly rising incidence of breast cancer over the last decade gives a particular timeliness to *Estrogen and Breast Cancer*. Carol Ann Rinzler focuses on the most important sources of estrogens that are under the control of women: oral contraceptives and estrogen replacement therapy. From her description of the discovery of estrogens, their rise and fall through the menstrual cycle, and their relation to breast cancer, the reader will gain a clear understanding of the many pieces of evidence that confirm the link between estrogens and breast cancer.

Breast cancer is caused by estrogens, both those produced by the body during the reproductive years and those added through the use of oral contraceptives and replacement hormone therapy. The steady rise in the incidence of breast cancer from 1940 onward may reflect the parallel decline in the average age at menarche (the onset of menstrual periods), due in part to improved childhood nutrition and decreased frequency of major childhood illnesses, decreasing family size, and increasing levels of obesity among postmenopausal women. While estrogen is the proximate cause of breast cancer, these changes are more distal causes that are mediated through estrogen. Increases in alcohol consumption by women during the twentieth century have also contributed to the long-term rise in incidence. The more rapid rise in the incidence of breast cancer since 1980 (with an increase of up to four percent per year) may be attributed, in part, to increased detection with the use of screening mammography and to the more widespread use of estrogens.

At least 50 million women in the United States have used oral contraceptives since these drugs were introduced in 1960, and more than 10 million women were using them in 1988. The author elegantly summarizes a large body of scientific studies showing that current use of oral contraceptives is associated with an increased risk of breast cancer. Likewise, for studies of the link between breast cancer and the estrogen replacement therapy used by postmenopausal women, the author sets forth a clear, concise, and insightful history. Again, the evidence overwhelmingly shows that current use increases the risk of breast cancer. For women over sixty, the use of replacement estrogens doubles the risk of breast cancer.

Through this carefully researched book, Ms. Rinzler has assembled an important synopsis of the history of the scientific inquiry and public debate surrounding the use of estrogens in oral contraceptives and replacement therapy. Overall themes of the book include:

- the "medicalization" of the stages of the life cycle;
- the burden of contraception and body image; and
- the lock on research and treatment frames that keep "medicine" moving in one direction rather than encouraging the exploration of multiple approaches.

The social assumptions about women that underlie the first two themes find expression in political priorities and bear on a fourth theme:

• the scientific silences that are tolerated in the medical community.

This book is a valuable resource and should be essential reading for all women who consider using oral contraceptives and estrogen replacement therapy as well as for those who will prescribe these treatments.

Ms. Rinzler concludes her book with "An Agenda for Women," in which she defines a blueprint for the future. While she notes that balancing risks and benefits remains a thorny problem, she identifies several key questions that may help women who use estrogens to do so more safely. She advocates streamlined regulatory processes with more information included in the packaging of all products that contain estrogen, increased efforts to identify women who are at risk when they take estrogen, and greater research into the development of new and safer forms of The Pill. Finally, she offers some sound advice: Use hormone replacement therapy only when necessary, and use safe alternatives to chemical contraception and hormone replacement therapy whenever possible.

To fulfill this agenda, we must keep our focus on the rising burden of breast cancer and on alternative approaches to the prevention of heart disease (and perhaps osteoporosis) that rely not on drugs but on individual changes, such as an increase in the role of exercise in women's lives, and on broader social changes, such as an end to selective marketing of tobacco to women. The assumption that breast cancer is the "cost" of preventing heart disease and osteoporosis must be challenged. Balancing of risks and benefits of multiple endpoints, including heart disease and osteoporosis, is complex; to date, sufficient emphasis has not been placed on the quality of life. Greater knowledge of the impact of prevention strategies (both pharmacologic and nonpharmacologic) on women's quality of life will better inform the tradeoffs that must be made.

Prevention efforts that take into account the social response to menopause, that challenge the underlying assumption by physicians that menopause is a disease, and that explore alternative ways to think about women who are aging will allow us to move beyond the medical model and so more carefully assess the need for replacement estrogens and oral contraceptives. Such a shift in focus is imperative if we are to lessen the burden of illness that breast cancer places on women.

Graham A. Colditz, M.D.
Associate Professor of Medicine,
Harvard Medical School
Project Director, Nurses
Health Study

# Acknowledgments

The author is indebted to the following people for their contributions to the writing of this book. George Berkovitz helped me translate statistics into language anyone can understand. Dana Points took the time to dig up a clipping I needed at a difficult turn in the manuscript. Martin S. Begun made it possible for me to use the wonderful library at New York University Medical Center. My mother, Rosalind Rinzler, unearthed a 25-year-old copy of *Feminine Forever*. Rica Rinzler and Myrna Egeth listened to my complaints without complaining. Linda R. Troiano encouraged me to begin to write about estrogen and breast cancer for a small article in *Good Housekeeping*. Graham Colditz, I. Craig Henderson, Robert Hoover, Edward F. Lewison, Malcolm Pike, and a number of epidemiologists and cancer experts were gracious enough to read and comment on this manuscript. Finally, my agent, Phyllis Westberg, and my editor at Macmillan, Natalie Chapman, had sufficient grace under author-induced pressure to keep things moving smoothly at all times.

# Introduction

Even when you know what you are going to see, the numbers are shocking.

In 1940, cancer of the breast was already the most common cancer among American women. There were about 59 cases a year for every 100,000 women in the country; the lifetime risk was 1-in-20.

By 1990, the incidence of cancer of the uterus and cancer of the stomach, which had been the second and third most common cancers among American women in 1940, had gone down by as much as 70 percent, but the incidence of breast cancer was 80 percent higher.

Today, there are 105 cases of breast cancer for every 100,000 women in the United States. The lifetime risk among women who live to be eighty-five is 1-in-9; adding women who live longer brings it to 1-in-8. The number of new cases each year, which until 1982 had been rising at an annual rate of 1.1 percent, is now going up nearly four times as fast, 4.3 percent a year.

Because breast cancer, like most other cancers, is most common among older people, it is safe to assume that at least some of the increase in incidence and risk is due simply to the fact that there are now more older women in this country. Between 1940 and 1990, the life expectancy for American women went up thirteen years; between 1960 and 1990, the number of women older than forty-four increased 64 percent.

More efficient early detection has also pushed the numbers up. For example, in 1973, there were 79.8 new cases reported for every 100,000 women. The following year, when Betty Ford and Margaretta "Happy" Rockefeller were diagnosed with breast cancer within three weeks of each other and thousands of women went to their doctors for mammograms, there was a sudden jump up to 91 reported cases per 100,000 women. But by 1975 it was back down to 84.6 per 100,000.

But after you adjust the statistics to reflect an older population and rejigger them to account for early detection, there is still a sustained upward swing in the incidence of breast cancer and in an individual woman's risk of the disease, a risk that is rising faster every year.

It took twenty years, from 1940 to 1960, for an American woman's lifetime risk of breast cancer to go from 1-in-20 to 1-in-14. It took another eleven years, from 1977 to 1988, for it to go to 1-in-10. But only two years later it was 1-in-9. Today it is 1-in-8.

Cancer of the breast is not a contagious disease, but many people understandably bend the semantic line to call what is happening here an epidemic.

The question is: What is causing it?

Experts have suggested a wide variety of reasons, chief among them a high-fat diet, a genetic predisposition, and exposure to environmental toxins. Eventually, there may be evidence to prove that one of these—or something else that no one has yet thought of—is indeed the culprit. But right now the clearest epidemiological paper trail leads in another direction, to another cause.

This book proposes to follow that trail, to explore the possibility that a major, avoidable, direct cause of America's fifty-year-old breast cancer epidemic has been our growing exposure to estrogen in the form of oral contraceptives and post-menopausal estrogen replacement therapy (ERT).

This is not a story with clear-cut heroes and villains. Nor is it an absolute condemnation of The Pill and ERT. All medicines have risks as well as benefits. The intelligent doctor and patient will make sure the trade-offs are observed, which, in this case, means prescribing hormones only for the women who really need them.

Because that hasn't always happened, the history of female hormone therapy in this country has sometimes seemed, in the words of Sidney Wolfe, director of the Washington-based Public Citizen Health Research Group, to be a tale of "false promises, disregard for scientific evidence and the wishful thinking of women and their doctors that all female health problems might vanish with the magic of pills. It is a story of well-meaning doctors eager to please, and of women too easily sold the wonders of pharmaceutical cures."

Above all, it is a story of what happened when the magic failed and the cure began to kill.

Breast cancer is the most feared cancer and the one most often discovered by the patient herself. It is the cancer which has given rise to the most articles in medical journals, the one for which most biopsies and most X-ray examinations are performed. It is the cancer treated most controversially and most radically. It is the cancer which involves the most surgical operations, the most radiation therapy, the most chemotherapy, and the most hormone therapy. It is the most costly cancer to the patient in financial terms. Finally it is the most prolific cancer in sheer quantity of neoplastic tissue produced by human beings.

—ROALD GRANT, M.D.
FIRST NATIONAL CONFERENCE ON BREAST CANCER
WASHINGTON, D.C., MAY 1969

I swear by Apollo the physician, by Aesculapius, Hygeia, and Panacea, and I take to witness all the gods, all the goddesses, to keep according to my ability and judgment the following Oath . . . I will prescribe regimen for the good of my patients according to my judgment and ability and never do harm to anyone.

—FROM THE PHYSICIANS' OATH ATTRIBUTED TO
HIPPOCRATES OF COS, CA. 460–400 B.C.

# Estrogen

# chapter 1

# The Female Principle

## *The Mysterious Ovary*

From the moment of conception, our genes and chromosomes make us either male or female, but it takes a while for our bodies to catch up.

As late as the twelfth week of pregnancy, when the fetus already has arms and legs and fingers and toes, the genitals are visible simply as swellings that will eventually become either penis or vagina. It takes until the twentieth week for the gonads (sex glands) to become ovaries if the fetus is female and testicles if it is male. Then, at some point between weeks twenty-eight to thirty-two, a month after all the vital organs of the body have been formed and the fetus has developed eyebrows and lashes as well as characteristic ridges on the palms of the hands and the soles of the feet, the male gonads descend into the scrotum. The female gonads, now ovaries, remain inside the body.

Because the testicles are outside the body, it was easy to figure out that they had a direct role to play in the development and function of a man's body. Well before there was any real scientific understanding of reproductive physiology, ordinary people knew that these organs were in some way responsible for a man's "maleness." Removing the testicles before a boy reached puberty kept him from developing an adult male's deep voice, strong ropy muscles, beard and body hair. In adulthood, the loss of the testicles virtually eliminated sexual desire and potency. Devotees of the Phoenician goddess Astarte and the Greek goddess Cybele are said to have practiced self-castration to prove their single-minded devotion to their deity. On a more practical level, ancient rulers such as the Persian emperor Cyrus used castration to create eunuchs who could guard the bedchambers of the palace without being tempted. In the year A.D. 325, the Council of Nicaea barred voluntary castrates from the priesthood, but the custom was revived in the sixteenth century to produce pure soprano voices for the choirs of the Roman Catholic church, only to be outlawed finally in Western nations through an edict published by Pope Clement XIV in 1770.

The effects of the ovaries were less obvious, almost certainly because the ovaries themselves were less obvious, tucked away deep inside a woman's body. The only way to observe them directly would have been through either dissection or surgery. But for centuries the first was forbidden by a religious belief in the resurrection of the entire body after death, and without anesthetics or an understanding of how to prevent infections, the second was impractical.

---

**Looking into the body.** Until the middle of the sixteenth century, virtually everything people knew about their own internal organs came from the work of the Greek-born physician Galen, who based his observations of anatomy on the dissections of dead animals. Alas, this produced a raft of misconceptions such as the idea that the human breastbone was built in segments, like an ape's, and the notion that the human uterus was composed of two hornlike chambers, like a dog's.

The first step toward an accurate, firsthand experience of the internal anatomy of the human body (including, of course, the female reproductive tract) occurred in 1543, when Andreas Vesalius, a young Flemish medical student at the University of Padua in Italy, published *De humani corporis fabrica* ("The Construction of the Human Body") based on his own dissection of a human body.

Vesalius' publication of his book was an act of physical, as well as intellectual, courage. His observations were a challenge not only to the medical establishment but to the theological authorities too. The Roman Catholic church considered dissection a sin; but by 1556, that had changed. The Church relented, declaring dissection of human cadavers useful to mankind. Gradually, anatomical study became permissible, although for the next several hundred years it was almost always performed on the bodies of executed criminals, mostly male.

The dissection of male bodies did little to advance the understanding of uterus and ovaries, and not much to increase the skill of surgeons, because without adequate anesthesia an internal operation was still a rare event. In fact, surgery was pretty much limited to amputation, the repair of wounds on the surface of the body, and an occasional cesarean delivery. What's more, without reliable antiseptic procedures, even a patient who came out of one of these operations alive was likely to succumb to infection afterward.

Then, on October 16, 1846, Boston dentist William Morton, who had learned to perform painless dentistry by anesthetizing his patients with ether, was invited to Massachusetts General Hospital to anesthetize a patient for the world's first painless surgical procedure. Afterward the astonished surgeon, John Warren, is reported to have turned to the assemblage and said: "Gentlemen, this is no humbug."

The next advance came in 1865 when Louis Pasteur

proposed his germ theory, the idea that infection was spread by microscopic organisms, which meant that if you removed (or killed) the organisms you could prevent infection. It took a while for surgeons to get the hang of it. In Vienna, Ludwig Ignaz Philipp Semmelweis was virtually driven out of medicine for the "crime" of attempting to convince doctors to wash their hands in chlorinated lime before moving from one obstetrical patient to the next, but infection control became the norm after 1866 when English surgeon Joseph Lister published his seminal paper entitled "On the Antiseptic Principle in the Practices of Surgery."

Lister did not invent antiseptics. People had been using wine (alcohol) and vinegar (acetic acid) to clean and dress wounds ever since the time of the ancient Greeks. Lister's great contribution was inventing the "antiseptic method": sterilizing instruments and dressings before surgery began, washing surgeons' hands and patients' skin in antiseptic solution, using surgical masks to cover the noses and mouths of the operating team so they did not spray germs into the air, and resterilizing instruments once the surgery was finished.

Now, with internal surgery safer and more common, surgeons operating at a more leisurely pace were beginning to expand their understanding of a woman's body.

These early explorers took some spectacularly wrong turns. In 1872, for example, American surgeon Robert Battey invented "female castration"—the removal of the ovaries—as a "cure" for menopause. His operation was endorsed by others, including American gynecologist Andrew Currier, who warned his colleagues to be sure to do a complete job: fallopian tubes and uterus, as well as both ovaries.

But sometimes they were headed in the right direction. By the end of the century they knew that something in the ovary itself affected the functions of the female body, and that while female castration could not cure menopause, removing the ovaries of a woman with breast cancer might slow the course of her disease. In 1896, Glasgow surgeon Sir George Beatson published a report to the British medical journal *Lancet* detailing a series of operations in which women with breast cancer were successfully treated by ovariectomy. "Eight months after castration," he wrote, "all vestiges of [the breast] cancer disappeared."

## *Finding the Female Hormones*

From earlier studies, mostly in animals, doctors were aware that ductless glands such as the thyroid and the adrenals secreted substances called hormones (from the Greek word *hormon*, which means "to excite"), and that these secretions played an important role in bodily processes. For example, extracts of the thyroid gland relieved the symptoms of hypothyroidism (an undersecretion of thyroid hormones). It was reasonable to assume that the ovaries also produced substances that affected body functions. As early as 1896, even before they knew what estrogen was, doctors were prescribing for "female problems," including menopause, extracts made of tissue from the ovaries of cows. In 1900, Viennese gynecologist Emil Knauer discovered that transplanting ovaries into female animals whose own gonads had been removed could reverse symptoms that were similar to what happened to women going through menopause.

But nobody yet could identify the active principle in the ovarian tissue. Certainly none of the doctors who adopted Beatson's procedure and were busily removing ovaries from women with breast cancer really knew why this helped their patients. Their justification for the operation was simple: About 50 percent of the time, taking out a breast cancer patient's ovaries made her tumor shrink.

Then, in 1923, the search for the active chemical in ovarian extracts moved a giant step forward when two American researchers, Edgar Allen, M.D., and Edward A. Doisy, M.D., devised a way to measure the "strength" of extracts prepared from the ovaries of laboratory rats. This involved simply observing the changes that occurred in the cells in the vaginal walls of the rats who were given the extracts. The "stronger" the extract, the greater the cell changes. Two years later, a "female principle" was identified in the blood of several different species of female animals, then in the urine of sows in heat, and finally in the urine of menstruating women. What they found was the primary female hormone—actually a group of related substances. They named it estrogen from *oistros/oestrus*, the Greek and Roman words for "frenzy," and *gen*, the Greek and Latin root for "begin."

Within a year, researchers knew that the amount of estrogen in a woman's urine rose and fell with her menstrual cycle. In 1928, German obstetrician-gynecologist Bernhardt Zondek reported that pregnant women excreted large amounts of estrogen in their urine, and soon it was clear that estrogen levels remained high throughout pregnancy and declined dramatically at menopause.* In 1929, estrone, the first estrogen to be crystallized in a laboratory, was isolated from the urine of pregnant women. Fourteen years later, Edward Doisy, one of the researchers to perform this feat, was awarded a Nobel Prize for medicine.

---

* Zondek is perhaps best known as the co-developer of the Aschheim-Z (Zondek) pregnancy test in which, contrary to common belief, the rabbit *always* dies. To perform the test, the doctor injected the rabbit with urine or blood from a woman suspected to be pregnant. The rabbit was then sacrificed a few days later. If the woman was pregnant, her hormone-laden urine or blood would change the appearance of the rabbit's ovaries, making them look as though the animal itself was pregnant.

## *What Estrogen Does*

The body makes three principal forms of estrogen: estrone, estradiol, and estriol.* Estradiol, the most potent, most plentiful estrogen, is secreted by the ovaries, the testes, the placenta, and the cortex (outer covering) of the adrenal glands. Estrogens are also produced by the conversion of steroid chemicals in body fat, which, along with the adrenal cortex, is considered the major source of estrogen production in men and post-menopausal women.

After puberty and before menopause, a woman who is having normal menstrual cycles secretes approximately 70 to 500 micrograms (mcg) estradiol a day, depending on the phase of the menstrual cycle.† Estradiol is metabolized in the liver where it is converted to estrone, a much less active estrogen, which is eventually excreted in urine. Estrone, which is also secreted by the placenta and the testes and produced by conversion of steroid hormones in body fat, is metabolized to estriol, another less potent estrogen, usually the most plentiful estrogen found in urine.

Estrogen is vital to being female, but it is not exclusive to a woman's body. In the beginning, all gonads are gender neutral. Whether they become ovaries or testes is decided when the X and Y chromosomes that make a person male (XY) or female (XX) begin to exert their influence on the growing fetus. Throughout life, both ovaries and testes retain the ability to secrete both male hormones, which are known collectively as androgens, and the female hormone estrogen. Overall, however, a man's body produces more androgens (the most important of which is testosterone); a woman's, more estrogen. It is this balance among the sex hormones,

---

* In scientific terms, the word *estrogen* usually refers specifically to a form of estradiol called 17-*b* estradiol.

† A milligram (mg) is 1,000th of a gram. A microgram (mcg) is 1,000th of a milligram.

not the absence of one or the other, that makes a person male or female.

In a woman's body, estrogen rules sexual development and sexuality. At puberty, hormones secreted by the pituitary gland, which is located in the brain, stimulate a woman's ovaries to produce estrogen. The estrogen, in turn, stimulates the development of her breasts, the maturation of her reproductive tract, and the appearance of her secondary sexual characteristics—pubic hair, underarm hair, and pigmentation of the nipples.

Estrogen also regulates the menstrual cycle, triggering the release of an egg from the ovaries each month. When the egg is released, the corpus luteum—the tissue created from the wall of the sac in which the egg was held—begins to secrete progesterone (*pro* = for, *gest* = bear; i.e., pregnancy). This second female hormone thickens and firms the lining of the uterus, nourishing the extra blood vessels needed to supply the fetus. It also prevents the release of another egg, thus preventing two pregnancies in the same month.* After ovulation, as progesterone levels rise, estrogen levels fall, and if a fertilized egg does not implant in the thickened wall of the uterus, the relatively high amounts of progesterone in the body stimulate the shedding of the endometrial tissue we recognize as menstrual bleeding. When that occurs, estrogen levels start to climb again, and the cycle begins anew.

Throughout her reproductive years, estrogen seems to protect a woman against coronary artery disease. For unknown reasons, it does not offer the same courtesy to men.

---

* *Progesterone* is a natural female hormone produced by the body. Chemicals that act like progesterone are commonly called *progestogens*. The overall name for the group of chemicals that includes both progesterone and progestogens is *progestins*. Progestins may be derived from plants or synthesized in the laboratory from other steroid hormones such as testosterone. Natural progesterone inhibits some of the effects of estrogen, so it is called an antiestrogen. Some synthetic progestins mimic some of the effects of estrogen and androgens.

From 1970 to 1973, the National Heart, Lung and Blood Institute, a division of the National Institutes of Health (NIH), sponsored a study conducted by the Coronary Drug Project Research Group in which men at risk for heart disease were given daily doses of estrogen in the hope that if estrogen protected pre-menopausal women, it might also protect men. Like a similar experiment in the 1960s, this one was a dismal failure. Within a year, researchers found that men taking estrogen had more, not fewer, heart attacks. So they lowered the doses, only to find that while there was no longer an effect on a man's risk of heart attack, even very small doses of estrogen could still shrink his testicles, enlarge his breasts, and reduce his sex drive, sometimes to the point of impotence.

After menopause, estrogen demonstrates its power over a woman's body by virtue of what happens as ovarian function declines and estrogen production slows (but never entirely ceases). She may have hot flushes, her skin and the tissue of her vaginal walls dry and thin, her bones become more porous and fragile, and her risk of heart attack rises, eventually, after age sixty-five, coming close to that of a man. As they grow older, men also secrete smaller amounts of sex hormones, and very late in life, as the secretion of sex hormones continues to decline for both men and women, a man's facial hair thins, a woman's grows darker and heavier; scalp and body hair thin; men become less muscular, women less plump; and at the end, the sexes come to resemble each other, just as they did when they were infants before the rising hormone tides of puberty made them recognizably adult men and women.

But that is not the point of this story. What interests us here is that the availability of purified estrogen, followed by the isolation of progesterone in 1934 and the male hormone testosterone in 1935, made it temptingly possible to manipulate a woman's hormonal balance. If the discomfort a woman experienced at menopause could be alleviated by estrogen, then why not simply give her the medicine she required?

It was so reasonable a proposition that soon the idea began to percolate up through the medical community that *all* of the natural phases of a woman's reproductive life—menstruation, fertility, pregnancy, as well as menopause—could be similarly relieved, cured, or improved by keeping a woman's estrogen level high every day of her life for as long as she lived.

It was a miscalculation of potentially tragic proportions.

# chapter 2

# Medicine for Menopause 1930–1960

## How Menopause Became a Disease

There are three natural stages in a woman's reproductive life. First come the years from birth to puberty; next, the years from menarche (the first menstrual period) to menopause, years when she is fertile and capable of becoming pregnant; third, the years after menopause, when she is sexually mature but no longer fertile.

Historically, the first stage of a woman's life, her childhood, is the only time when nobody calls her names. Menstruation, the very symbol of female fertility and adulthood, has often been described as "the curse," the strange bleeding without injury that set women apart from men and made them unacceptable, unclean. Infertility was a curse of a different sort, like the pain of childbirth, a punishment of the gods.

But menopause was worse. In her landmark text, *Psychology of Women: A Psychoanalytic Interpretation,* psychiatrist Helene Deutsch called it a "partial death." A 1980 best-seller on "women's problems," written by gynecologist Penny Wise Budoff, M.D., who advocated the use of estrogen to relieve menopausal symptoms, makes clear her astonishment that as late as the 1980s: "It was considered a *natural* event when the ovaries failed [and menopause] was considered *natural* [italics added], desirable, and even good for our health.''

This view of menopause as unnatural, a partial death, is not unique to these two women. Most American physicians keep a copy of *The Merck Manual* in their office library to provide a fast and handy review of current medical opinion. The first edition of this compact but comprehensive reference book (known as *Merck's Manual* until the sixth edition in 1934) appeared in 1898. Subsequent editions have followed every six to ten years since. In each edition the entry on menopause reflects a specific moment in the evolution of the medical profession's attempt to diagnose and treat as an illness what is nothing more (or less) than a normal part of every healthy woman's life.

In 1911, when 82 percent of the people in the United States were younger than forty-five and menopause of little serious concern, *Merck's* description was simple and straightforward: "The period in a woman's life when menstruation comes to an end." By 1923, however, menopause had mutated into "a physiological condition bordering on the pathological." In 1934, the editors calmed a bit, suggesting that women be "impresssed with the necessary philosophical tolerance of a physiological process and assisted to maintain mental and physical stability." In 1940, menopause was coupled with "hypo-ovarianism" and formally declared a disease. Ten years later, it was linked with "primary ovarian deficiency" and abnormally early puberty into an unhealthy triad under the heading "Ovarian dysfunction." In 1977, it became a "common gynecological problem," right alongside pelvic pain, vaginal infections, inflammatory disease, and PMS. It was still there in the 1992 edition.

So long as menopause was regarded as an "illness," physicians quite naturally sought a "cure," even though many argued that for most women—a number some put as high as 60 percent—the symptoms of menopause were temporary and manageable. Hot flushes were likely to wane after a year or two, lotions and creams could moisten dry skin, over-the-counter vaginal lubricants could make intercourse more comfortable, and the emotional ups-and-downs would eventually even out.

Others, however, were swayed by the descriptions in *Merck* ("pathological condition," "deficiency," "dysfunction," and "gynecological problem") and by their own patients' reports of physical discomfort along with the emotional distress caused by a belief that they were aging and sexually unattractive. Given all this, it would be a rare physician indeed who would ignore the possibility of a "cure," especially when the suggested remedy was a perfectly natural substance, one found in every woman's body.

In its first edition, *Merck* had recommended pills containing ovarian tissue from cows for menopausal women. These products, sold under names such as Ovaraden and Ovariin, were used along with such old-fashioned therapies as "attention to the emunctories [organs that carry off waste], avoidance of worry, increased rest, [a] simple diet with moderate nitrogenous content [and] moderate exercise in the open." If none of these worked, there were always salt baths, sedatives, and cannibis, which (in 1934) *Merck* called "worthy of a trial."

The introduction of purified natural estrogen pushed the crude ovarian extracts out of the gynecological medicine chest. Within a few years after the first American woman got the first shot of estrogen in 1931, there were a dozen different brands of the female hormone on the market, to be given as injections two or three times a week for two or three months until the menopausal patient reached "endocrine equilibrium"—meaning no return of symptoms once the injections stopped.

As previously noted, estrogen and progesterone activate important phases of the menstrual cycle. The cyclic high level of estrogen stimulates the release of the egg from the ovary; the subsequent high level of progesterone triggers the shedding of the endometrium that produces menstrual bleeding. Thus, estrogen injections were soon prescribed along with progesterone to relieve painful menstruation or to "bring on" a delayed first period or to remedy missing periods blamed on hormonal imbalance. They were also used as a remedy for chlorosis (the "green sickness," which may have been an early name for iron deficiency anemia), nervousness, angina pectoris, epilepsy, and osteomalacia (the adult version of rickets, a softening of the bones due to lack of calcium).

Injectable estrogen certainly proved to be more effective than dried ovarian extract, but it wasn't perfect. Natural estrogens do not dissolve in water. To be used as an injection, they had to be mixed with oils, and the oily liquid tended to leak out at the injection site. To prevent this, physicians in the late 1930s were told to point the hypodermic needle downward into the patient's buttocks and to stick on an adhesive plaster for a day or so. Then, in 1938, Hans H. Inhoffen and a group of chemists at Schering solved that problem when they discovered that by replacing one hydrogen atom on the estradiol molecule with a group of atoms called an ethinyl radical, they could make a new compound that had potent estrogenic activity when taken by mouth in pill form. That same year, British steroid chemist Sir Charles Dodds created diethylstilbestrol (DES), the first synthetic estrogen. It, too, could be made into a pill.

## Side Effects

In the early 1930s the only law regulating prescription and patent medicines in the United States was a truth-in-labeling code that prohibited the sale of "misbranded" products. Manufacturers had to tell customers what was in the product and could not lie about what the drug could do. But it wasn't until 1938—the year ethinyl estradiol and DES appeared, nine years after estrogen was isolated—that Congress passed the first law requiring drug manufacturers to test a product for safety before putting it on the market.

As a result, hormones had been introduced into medicine without any formal testing, and as they grew ever more popular, the only way to tell whether they were also safe and effective was to watch what happened to women who used them.

Every physician knows that any drug powerful enough to cure is also powerful enough to cause side effects. It was inevitable that that would happen with estrogen. But when the hormone caused vaginal bleeding or sore breasts or "nervous tension," doctors simply prescribed another hormone, this time the male hormone testosterone, either alone or in tandem with the estrogen.

It didn't solve the problem. Testosterone was bad news for menopausal women. Even small amounts could be masculinizing. Women who used it were distressed to find their facial hair growing darker and thicker, the hair on their head thinning, their voices deepening to a masculine timbre, and acne, the curse of the adolescent hormone storm, blooming on their middle-aged faces. As a result, testosterone soon fell from favor as a menopausal remedy. The market for post-menopausal estrogen replacement therapy (ERT) continued to expand quietly through the 1950s, driven by the undeniable fact that women with hot flushes and vaginal dryness usually felt better when they took estrogen.

This created a loyal but still relatively small band of women who continued to use estrogen at menopause, private patients getting estrogen from gynecologists or family doctors.* Then, starting around 1941, there was a new and growing audience for estrogens: pregnant women taking DES on the theory that because estrogen levels rise naturally during pregnancy, the extra estrogen would make the fetus healthier and reduce to zero the risk of miscarriage.

---

**Estrogens for pregnant women.** Miscarriage (also known as spontaneous abortion) is generally defined as the loss of the fetus sometime before the twentieth to twenty-sixth week of pregnancy. Approximately 1-in-6 pregnancies are known to end in spontaneous abortion, but the number may be higher because a spontaneous abortion that occurs before the end of the fourth week may never have been noticed as a pregnancy. In most cases, spontaneous abortion is due to a defect in the fetus that makes it unlikely to survive. However, a woman who experiences three or more spontaneous abortions in a row ("habitual abortion") is likely to be suffering from a physical problem such as diabetes, kidney disease, thyroid disease, or an anatomical abnormality of the uterus or cervix that cannot resist the downward pressure of the expanding uterus.

In 1941, based on the observation that women who suffered a spontaneous abortion were likely to have lower blood levels of estrogen than were women whose pregnancies proceeded uneventfully to term, a husband and wife team named George and Olive Smith (he a gynecologist, she an epidemiologist) at the Free Hospital for Women in Boston, decided that estrogen for the mothers would protect the fetuses. The estrogen they chose was diethylstilbestrol (DES).

---

* As late as 1967, one prominent estrogen enthusiast estimated that there were only about 14,000 "sexually restored, post-menopausal women" in the United States, an admittedly "puny fraction" of the millions waiting for help. The real number, though, may have been larger. There was no formal count of the women using ERT.

From 1943 through 1948, the Smiths prescribed DES to 632 pregnant women, 515 in Boston and another 117 in forty-eight other cities across the country where gynecologists were eager to cooperate by giving the pills to expectant mothers and watching to see what happened. The babies born to these women were described not just as healthy but as "grossly" more healthy than babies whose mothers hadn't taken DES. In 1949, the Smiths completed a second DES study. This time, 389 pregnant women who took DES were compared with 550 who did not. Again all the pregnancies, DES as well as non-DES, seemed normal. Again the Smiths said that the babies born to women who had taken DES seemed healthier; perhaps, they suggested, the drug "stimulated better placental function and hence bigger and healthier babies."

The use of DES by pregnant women expanded the market dramatically; some people estimate that as many as 4 million used DES between 1948 and 1961. By 1952 there was an estrogen for every taste, more than thirty different brands of injectable solutions, pills, ointments, suppositories, and nasal sprays. But the number of women known to be using estrogens for menopause was still in the tens of thousands, so even when you added in the expectant mothers, it was still a relatively limited audience.

It was not until 1960 that the first truly explosive demand for an estrogen product occurred. It was triggered by the introduction of the birth control pill, an event that led directly to the first round of serious estrogen damage.

# chapter 3

# Reproductive Remedies 1937–1960

## *Birth Control: Simple, Safe, Cheap*

To people active in the modern reproductive rights movement, the name Planned Parenthood conjures up the image of an organization whose primary goal is to protect a woman's right to reproductive freedom, including the right to a safe and legal abortion. But its founders had an agenda that was at once more simple and more universal: to prevent potentially disastrous world over-population.

Margaret Sanger, who established Planned Parenthood and founded the birth control movement in the United States, wanted a method of birth control acceptable to people from widely different cultures. "The world and almost our civilization for the next 25 years," Sanger wrote in 1950, "is going to depend on a simple, cheap, safe contraceptive." This new contraceptive had to satisfy the needs of women who found the diaphragm embarrassing because using it required them to touch their genitals, and those who could not rely on condoms because using them required a partner's cooperation, not always easily come by. A chemical contraceptive—a once-a-month injection or, better yet, a once-a-day pill—would be an elegant solution that would work as well in the underdeveloped areas of the world as in the sophisticated West.

In 1951, Sanger met with Gregory Goodman Pincus, scientific director of the Worcester Foundation for Experimental Biology in Massachusetts. At the time, Pincus headed up a team that included Min-Chueh Chang, an expert in the field of artificial insemination and sperm biology whom Pincus had brought to the United States from Cambridge in 1945. The two were working furiously to create a chemical contraceptive.

The site of the Pincus/Sanger meeting is uncertain (Pincus said he remembered Sanger coming to see him in Massachusetts; others remember his going to meet her in New York), but there is no doubt about what happened: Sanger impressed on Pincus her belief that in the future the real work in contraception would come from chemistry. Researchers at Pennsylvania State University had discovered in 1937 that both natural estrogen and natural progesterone could suppress the release of an egg from the ovary when administered to laboratory rabbits, a fact that led some scientists to call the hormone "nature's contraceptive."

Pincus left the meeting with the promise of $2,100 toward the cost of the first year's research into the value of the female hormone progesterone as the key to effective chemical birth control. Sanger's contribution was followed by a $40,000 down payment on a $125,000 donation from another birth control pioneer, Katherine McCormick, daughter-in-law of Cyrus McCormick, the inventor of the mechanical reaper, and then by a contribution from Sanger's Planned Parenthood Federation, which allowed Pincus and Chang to proceed with their studies.

At the same time, John Rock and his team of researchers at the Free Hospital for Women in Boston and the Reproductive Study Center just outside Boston in Brookline, were using the hormone to achieve exactly the opposite effect.

They were giving their patients progesterone in an attempt to cure female infertility.

---

**Infertility studies in Brookline.** John Rock, M.D., professor of gynecology at Harvard Medical School and head of the infertility clinic at the Free Hospital for Women in Boston, was a man with a definite sense of irony. A Roman Catholic, he would note in 1963, after the birth control pill was on the market, that "Life has a way now and then of mocking man's questionable designs. It must have amused the citizens of the Commonwealth of Massachusetts, with its rigid law against birth control, to discover that the first breakthrough in contraceptive technology in seventy-five years suffered and survived its labor pains in the environs of Worcester and Boston. Similarly, those who tend to see the drama of human fertility through one-dimension viewers must still be confused by the fact that the new birth-control pills may turn out to be a useful therapeutic agent in the prevention of repetitive miscarriage [which] have made many couples childless."

At Rock's Reproductive Study Center, eighty women who had not been able to conceive agreed to accept treatment with estrogen and progesterone, the natural hormones that Rock said "were known to be harmless." While they were taking the hormones, the women developed some of the symptoms of a true pregnancy. "They did not menstruate," Rock wrote in *The Time Has Come,* his 1963 book about the history of chemical contraception, "nor was ovulation detectable; the breasts and in some cases the uterus seemed to become larger." After treatment was stopped, the women began menstruating again, and within four months, thirteen of them were pregnant.

Next, Rock put a group of twenty-seven women on a three-month regimen of progesterone alone for twenty days of the menstrual cycle and no hormones at all the last week, a regime that once again produced withdrawal bleeding resembling a menstrual period. As the scientists at Pennsylvania State University had shown, progesterone, alone or with estrogen, did at least temporarily inhibit ovulation. But rather than accept this as proof that progesterone could not cure infertility, Rock interpreted this hormonally induced inhibition of ovulation as a sort of priming of the reproductive system that might lead to the return of ovulation. After all, once the treatment ended, four of his volunteers became pregnant.

At the time, researchers such as Pincus, Chang, and Rock were using natural progesterones obtained from the *corpus luteum* of various animals. The material was relatively scarce and using natural progesterone to stop ovulation required frequent injections of large amounts of the hormone, and these were as messy and unpleasant as the estrogen injections had been. The obvious solution was to give the progesterone in tablet form, but there was a problem. Early on, researchers who had tried what they regarded as reasonable doses of the hormone were unable to control ovulation. For a while, they thought the hormone was simply inactivated when taken by mouth. Instead, it turned out that enormous amounts of natural progesterone were required to inhibit ovulation when the hormone was given orally. When they realized the problem was dosage, the scientists increased the amount of progesterone they gave their patients. This worked.

Soon, Pincus was administering doses as high as 300 mg of the scarce natural progesterone obtained from various companies and laboratories. Rock was using doses ranging from 300 to 400 mg. It was effective, but the quantities required were so enormous that there simply was not enough natural progesterone available to make a long-term, large-scale experiment possible.

Clearly, the ultimate solution to the dilemma was to find

progesterone-like chemicals in nature or to manufacture synthetic ones in the laboratory. Until that happened, contraceptive research would proceed more slowly than anyone wanted.

---

**Synthesizing progesterones.**    The first step toward creating an adequate supply of synthetic progesterone was to look for analogous chemicals in plants. The search led to the identification of diosgenin, a substance whose molecular structure is only slightly different from that of natural progesterone.

Diosgenin, which is found in Mexican yams, is more potent than progesterone, so it is effective in smaller doses. It was discovered by Russell E. Marker, a legendary but quirky man who had written a doctoral thesis and then failed to get his Ph.D. degree in chemistry from the University of Maryland because he refused to take a required course in physical chemistry (he said it was boring). Parke-Davis, the pharmaceutical company that supported Marker's early work in progesterone synthesis, was not interested in his discovery of diosgenin. Neither were any of the other major drug companies, so in January 1944, Marker joined with Emeric Somlo and Federico Lehmann, the owners of a Mexican company, Laboratorios Hormona, to form a new company called Syntex (from *Syn*thesis and M*exi*co). Marker left Syntex the following year, but the drive to mass-produce synthetic progesterones for oral contraceptives and/or a fertility drug took a quantum leap in 1949 when steroid chemist Carl Djerassi joined the staff at Syntex. Within three years, in April 1952, Djerassi submitted to an annual meeting of the American Chemical Society a paper on the synthesis of a progesterone-like chemical known generically as norethisterone but called norethindrone in the United States.

Soon afterward, Djerassi sent a supply of norethindrone to

Roy Hertz, M.D., Ph.D., at the National Institutes of Health in Washington. Hertz became the first person to give the crystalline powder to laboratory rabbits. Then he gave it to other laboratory animals and finally to three patients enrolled in a study at the Clinical Center of the National Institute of Child Health and Human Development. The study was designed to evaluate the synthetic hormone's ability to control menstrual irregularities. Djerassi's new progestin turned out to be six to eight times more powerful than natural progesterone and clearly effective by mouth.

For two years, Syntex's patent on Djerassi's norethindrone molecule gave the company a monopoly on synthetic progesterone-like compounds. In effect, that also gave Syntex a strong hold on the production of any oral contraceptives. Then, in 1955, a year after Djerassi printed a full report on norethindrone in the *Journal of the American Chemical Society,* G.D. Searle filed a patent for a similar molecule, a synthetic progesterone-like compound called norethynodrel. Syntex cried foul and suggested that Searle had pirated its research. Searle insisted that it had been funding progestin research since 1951, the year Syntex filed its patent. In the end, nobody sued. Searle, which quickly created a norethynodrel oral contraceptive, began to call itself the inventor of The Pill, even going so far as to actually discuss trademarking the name, The Pill, but they never followed through on it. Both companies continued to produce progesterones and to compete for the new contraceptive research business in the race to be first with a usable pill.*

At the same time, back in Massachusetts, Pincus and Chang, who were convinced of progesterone's value as a

* Today, Syntex continues to make and market synthetic hormones as well as oral contraceptives (Brevicon, Norinyl, Tri-Norinyl) and a variety of other products. In 1968 the company was awarded a patent on naproxen, the second nonsteroidal anti-inflammatory drug. (Ibuprofen, the first, preceded naproxen by four years.)

contraceptive, wrote to a number of drug companies requesting supplies of synthetic progestins. Soon Chang had fifteen different ones with which to work. Twelve were discarded as less active than natural progesterone. Two—Syntex's norethindrone and Searle's norethynodrel—proved useful. (A third, Searle's norethandrolone, turned out to be more active than progesterone but not as active as norethindrone and norethynodrel; Searle subsequently marketed it as a body-building steroid.)

Pincus and Chang tried norethindrone and norethynodrel on rabbits and rats and then began to give it to small groups of women volunteers. The regimen was simple. After a month's observation to be certain that they were ovulating normally, the women were each given one of the progestins daily from the fifth to the twenty-fifth days of the cycle after the menstrual flow began. Then the progestin was withdrawn and, as expected, although none of the women ovulated, they all experienced bleeding that resembled normal menstruation.

Rock, too, was using synthetic progestins in his studies. He gave his volunteers progestins for the first twenty days of the cycle and then withdrew them to allow withdrawal bleeding during the last week. Once again, five months after the treatment ended, patients began to get pregnant, which meant that Rock's studies, originally intended to find a cure for infertility, were actually confirming Pincus and Chang's belief that progesterone was an effective contraceptive.

In 1955, Pincus and Chang went to the Fifth International Planned Parenthood Federation Conference in Tokyo with reports showing that the synthetic hormones' ability to control ovulation might make them valuable as chemical contraceptives. Strangely enough, nobody seemed terribly interested, although one scientist in attendance warned that the researchers needed "better evidence about the occurrence of side effects in human beings. It is not enough that we take presumed negative evidence about the lack of side effects from animal experiments to imply that no undesirable side effects would occur in human beings. There is an urgent need for prolonged observation before we draw any firm conclusions."*

## Testing The Pill

By 1956, one year before the Food and Drug Administration (FDA) approved the use of norethindrone and norethyno-drel for the treatment of menstrual disorders, it was time to find out once and for all if the progestins could also answer Margaret Sanger's call for a contraceptive pill.

At the time, a pharmaceutical company testing a new drug had to comply with the provisions of the 1938 Federal Food, Drug and Cosmetic Act, which required the FDA to approve a New Drug Application (NDA) testifying to the product's safety and effectiveness before it could be sold to the public.

The requirements of the NDA could be satisfied by sending samples of the new drug to doctors who would then give it to their patients and notify the company of any ill effects. All the manufacturer had to do was follow three simple guidelines:

1. Label the samples it was sending out to be tested: "Caution, new drug, limited by Federal law to investigational use."

* Pincus' influence on the development of chemical contraception extended far beyond the birth control pill. In 1957, a young French endocrinologist named Etienne-Emile Baulieu visited the United States on sabbatical and met with Pincus. Twenty-five years later, Baulieu, who credits Pincus as being one of the major influences on his personal and professional life, went on to develop the pill he calls "the unpregnancy drug," RU-486.

2. Ask each doctor or scientist to whom the drug was sent to sign a paper stating that he or she was qualified to test the drug.
3. Keep a list of the names of the scientists who got the drug and the size of the shipment each received.

There was no requirement to test the drug on animals before trying it on human beings or to find out whether it would cause cancer or birth defects. Nor was the doctor required to obtain permission ("informed consent") from the patients who got the drug.

When Pincus and Chang began to test their new birth control pill with a group of sixty women in Massachusetts, many of the subjects were medical students, but seven women, age eighteen to forty-three, were, as was the custom of the day, "volunteers" from a mental institution near Worcester—all classified as psychotics suffering from disorders such as mental depression or schizophrenia. Since none of the mental patients was having intercourse, the study was limited to figuring out how long their menstrual cycles were, monitoring the body temperature, doing biopsies of uterine tissue to analyze any changes in the endometrium, and analyzing hormones excreted by their urine.

As expected, the pills—either 40 mg norethindrone or 20 mg norethynodrel—did suppress ovulation, and none of the women seemed to suffer any ill effects. Pincus and Chang then picked sixteen psychotic men from the same institution to see how the pill affected men. In a five-and-a-half-month test, eight men got placebos, eight got norethynodrel, and some of the men who got the progestins were switched to the placebo for part of the time.

When the test ended, Pincus declared that the progestins had temporarily sterilized the men who took them, although as journalist Paul Vaughn, author of *The Pill on Trial* (1970), pointed out, it is hard to understand how he came to this conclusion since it was impossible to get sperm samples from these men. For one young man who had been on the progestins all the way through the test, the results were more severe: His testicles shrank and his prostate atrophied. But since no one planned to use progestin as a male contraceptive, the ability to shrink testicles and prostate was not considered a reason to stop testing them as contraceptives for women.

Pincus and Chang now decided to move on to full-scale field trials to which Rock, who had come to view hormones as a form of natural birth control that would be accepted by the Catholic church (he was, of course, wrong), would lend his expertise. The place they chose for the tests was Puerto Rico, specifically the Rio Piedras section of San Juan, where the study was to be carried out under the auspices of the Family Planning Association of Puerto Rico, an affiliate of Planned Parenthood.

"Numerous reasons have been given for this [choice]," Paul Vaughn wrote. "Pincus and Rock wanted to test the steroid regimen on poor and uneducated women. It was all very well to tell sophisticated Bostonians to take the pills once a day for a fixed number of days and then start again after a prescribed interval. The problem was whether this would work when the consumers were feckless and illiterate, and would not necessarily understand the method or remember to take the pills regularly. The ideal contraceptive, after all, would have to suit millions of women in the deprived countries [and] the trial should be carried out in a place where the population was reasonably stable but where the birthrate was high and the women most likely to be interested in a new form of contraceptive."

Today it would not be necessary for researchers to go outside the continental United States, but in the mid-1950s, the situation regarding birth control was analogous to that regarding abortion before the U.S. Supreme Court handed down its 1973 decision on *Roe* v. *Wade*. Several states, including Massachusetts, had laws on the books making it a crime to prescribe or dispense birth control.* Doing contraceptive research with a large population in one of the forty-eight states would definitely not be a comfortable situation for either scientist or subject, although later on, some smaller field trials were run in San Antonio, Los Angeles, and New York, among other places.

**The Pill in Puerto Rico.**   The pill that went to Puerto Rico was a progestin-only product containing Searle's norethynodrel. (Syntex's norethindrone had been disqualified after some tests on male rats suggested the drug had a slight masculinizing effect.) During the trials, though, it turned out that the progestin in the pills contained traces of estrogen-like chemicals. When the progestin was purified to get rid of the estrogens, the pill did not work as well. There was "breakthrough" bleeding in the middle of a woman's cycle and there was some question as to whether the pill, which contained only 10 mg norethynodrel, one-half the dose Pincus and Chang had used in 1954, was effectively controlling ovulation. So Searle put estrogen in the form of mestranol, a synthetic hormone, back in. The combination

---

* The widespread acceptance of contraception is relatively recent. In 1960, marital relations without the intent to conceive were declared by the General Assembly of the Southern Presbyterian church not to be sinful. It took another year for the National Council of Churches to endorse birth control as a means of family planning. In June 1965, the U.S. Supreme Court overturned an 1879 Connecticut law banning the use of contraceptives entirely, a law Supreme Court nominee Robert Bork did not consider unconstitutional. In Massachusetts, the law was changed in August 1966 to make contraception legal, but only for married people. Not until March 1972, when the U.S. Supreme Court overturned the Massachusetts law by a 4–3 decision, did it become legal for all Massachusetts adults, single as well as married, to use birth control.

of 10 mg norethynodrel and 0.15 mg mestranol was quickly patented under the trade name Enovid.*

The women who used the norethynodrel/mestranol pill for twenty days of the month experienced cycles that seemed wholly normal, complete with a period of menstrual-like flow at the end of the month. This was a definite plus because it convinced the volunteers that they were having regular periods, that they were not pregnant, and that their bodies were working normally.

There were, however, some disquieting ripples in the pond. Nearly 20 percent of the women taking The Pill developed at least one side effect. Some felt dizzy; some were sick to their stomachs; some had headaches, stomach pain, or diarrhea; and some had more than one of these symptoms at once.

The doctors in charge of the trials blamed these symptoms on the power of suggestion and set out to confirm their opinion with a quickly arranged second trial. They gave one group of women placebos and told them the pills were contraceptives. Along with the placebos, the women got a detailed warning about possible side effects. Sure enough, about 20 percent of them—the same percentage as in the original trial—developed side effects. A second group of women was given real birth control pills but no warnings of ill effects. Only 6 percent of these women reported problems, and this, the doctors said, proved that the side effects reported by women using oral contraceptives were mostly in the mind.

---

* In 1990, Wyeth-Ayerst introduced Norplant, a progestin-only implantable contraceptive. Norplant is more effective than the original progestin-only contraceptive pill because the implant delivers the hormone directly into the bloodstream in a low but steady concentration. Progesterone implants, it is interesting to note, had been used in the late 1930s by the researchers at Pennsylvania State University who first documented progesterone's ability to inhibit ovulation in laboratory rabbits.

The argument sounds convincing, but there are catches in it. First, if a woman taking oral contraceptives was not told that her headache, upset stomach, and mild dizziness were related to the pills, she might not even mention them to her doctor. Second, if even major adverse effects were ignored, would anyone really be on the look-out for less severe ones? Barbara Seaman, author of *The Doctors' Case Against The Pill* (1969) and *Women and the Crisis in Sex Hormones* (1977), noted that the scientists did not even ask for autopsies on three women who died while they were participating in the trials.

In any event, when the Puerto Rican tests ended in February 1957, there was an armload of hopeful statistics. In what the researchers described as "47 patient years" of experience with The Pill, there had been minor upsets but no serious side effects. Most important, not a single woman who had taken The Pill as directed got pregnant while she was using it.

On May 9, 1960, based on the data from Puerto Rico, the FDA approved Searle's pill, known as Enovid-10 because it contained 10 mg norethynodrel, for use as an oral contraceptive. In the first year it was on sale, approximately 800,000 American women filled their first prescription for the estrogen/progestin pill.

Within months, many had come to regret their decision. For an unfortunate few, the problem would go beyond regret. It was a fatal error.

# chapter 4

# Problems with The Pill 1961–1962

## *What the Doctors Knew*

For years, doctors experimenting with estrogen for menopausal women had promoted the hormone as a safe, natural remedy for a disease called menopause, and the men who invented The Pill relied on the same argument to justify using hormones for contraception. In *The Time Has Come*, for example, John Rock wrote that birth control pills "merely serve as adjuncts to nature." Used properly, he said, they were "not very likely to disturb menstruation, nor do they mutilate any organ of the body, nor damage any natural process."

It sounded good, but it was at best disingenuous.

In 1959, while the FDA was still reviewing the data from Searle's Puerto Rican trials, a group of British medical experts set up a year-long clinical trial of oral contraceptives under the sponsorship of the Family Planning Association, an affiliate of the International Planned Parenthood Federation. The English tested two estrogen/progestin products, Enovid and Primilut N, and on Wednesday, March 30, 1960, forty-one days before the FDA gave G.D. Searle permission to market its oral contraceptive in the United States, the British turned thumbs down on both, saying that while birth control pills were effective in preventing pregnancy, they caused too many immediate side effects to be put into general use.

Reports of headaches, nausea, weight gain, and a general malaise—the very things the researchers in Puerto Rico had dismissed as imaginary—convinced the British not to release the original pill. Instead, they decided to begin testing oral contraceptives made with smaller amounts of hormones to see if there was a formula that could keep a woman from becoming pregnant without exposing her to debilitating side effects.

The FDA did not agree. Estrogens were effective medicine. They eased menopausal discomfort and prevented pregnancy. If every doctor who prescribed them knew that estrogens might make some women miserably uncomfortable, that didn't matter to the FDA. In the United States, the government, the public, and Sidney Wolfe's "well-meaning doctors eager to please" were so bedazzled by the possibility of a remedy for menopausal discomfort and a pill to prevent pregnancy that they chose to ignore the evidence placed before them.

Nonetheless, as soon as The Pill went on sale here, it became obvious that the British had been right.

---

**Higher doses, younger women, bigger risks.** The form of estrogen most commonly used for post-menopausal hormone replacement therapy was (and still is) conjugated estrogens (a mixture of natural compounds isolated from the urine of mares). Milligram for milligram, conjugated estrogens are less potent than the estrogens used in The Pill. The first oral contraceptives were high-estrogen products that also contained a synthetic progestin with some estrogen-like activity. Thus, women on The Pill were being hit with a double whammy. Not only were they getting a more potent estrogen with birth control pills than there had been in the products used to treat menopausal symptoms, but there was also more natural estrogen in their pre-menopausal bodies.

Women taking estrogen replacement therapy (ERT) were at a point in their lives where their natural production of estrogen was diminishing; women filling prescriptions for oral contraceptives were young, and their bodies were still secreting normal amounts of sex hormones. ERT replaced a "missing" hormone; birth control pills added large amounts of a potent synthetic estrogen to the body's own natural supply, bathing the tissues in a continual tide of surplus hormones.

The result of this sudden widespread introduction of relatively high-dose estrogen products into a younger, larger population was a round of estrogen-related side effects. Women taking The Pill complained of nausea, migraine headaches, blurred vision, and swollen breasts or abdomen, only to be told that these were "temporary," "reversible" symptoms that would disappear with longer pill use.

But the most frightening immediate side effect of The Pill was the threat of potentially life-threatening blood clots.

---

**The Pill and vascular disease.**    All the pill researchers, including Gregory Goodman Pincus and John Rock, knew that taking estrogen reduced the time it took for blood to clot, which meant that women using birth control pills had a higher risk of embolisms, but the mechanism remained unclear and none of the scientists thought it was important enough to worry about.

It took some time to see a trend developing. First, within months after The Pill went on sale in 1961, two young California women using oral contraceptives died of pulmonary embolism (blood clot in the lungs). A steady stream of reports on blood clots among pill-users began to flow into the G.D. Searle corporate headquarters and, in lesser numbers, to the FDA in Washington. Even though there was no proof of a direct connection between The Pill and the blood clots, by May 1962, the FDA was sufficiently disturbed to ask G.D. Searle to notify all physicians in the United States that taking Enovid might raise the risk of embolism.

For several months the company stalled. Then, on Saturday, August 4, the FDA finally ran out of patience and released to the newspapers a report stating that in the twelve months between September 1961 and August 1962, twenty-eight American women had developed blood clots believed to be caused by oral contraceptives. Six of the twenty-eight had died.

The following Tuesday, August 7, while the St. Louis county coroner was reported to be investigating the death of a woman who developed a massive blood clot in her lungs after taking Enovid for two weeks, the Planned Parenthood Federation of America issued a statement saying that none of the nearly 11,000 women who had received a prescription for oral contraceptives at their clinics had developed blood clots. The organization's medical director, Mary S. Calderone, M.D., made it clear Planned Parenthood would continue to dispense The Pill at its clinics in the United States.

That was not the case in Norway, where fewer than half the two hundred chemists' shops were actually carrying oral contraceptives. The government ordered Enovid off the market after four British women developed blood clots while using The Pill. In Japan, the government avoided the debate about the safety of birth control pills by making the laws regulating the use of hormones for contraception so restrictive that virtually nobody could use The Pill.*

---

* The Japanese have remained consistent in opposing the use of oral contraceptives. In March 1992, officials in the Health and Welfare Ministry, citing evidence of a growing number of cases of AIDS, announced that it would keep in place its longtime restrictions on birth control pills. The condom is still the most widely used method of contraception in Japan.

Finally, Searle capitulated. On August 8, 1962, FDA commissioner George F. Larrick secured the company's agreement to notify U.S. doctors about the increased risk of blood clots among pill users. But on August 16, Miguel E. Paniagua, medical director of the Family Planning Association of Puerto Rico, told a reporter that there had been no blood clots evident in his trials. One month later, when Searle convened a medical conference in Chicago to talk about blood clots and The Pill, its tone was less conciliatory.

In August, G.D. Searle had accepted the fact that some women using Enovid-10 had developed blood clots, but it disputed the cause and continued to deny any link between the two. It also took issue with the numbers. William Crosson, assistant medical director at Searle Laboratories, told *The New York Times* that in any given year you could expect 71 of every 100,000 women age twenty to forty-five to be hospitalized for thrombophlebitis (a blood clot in a vein). "Since about a million women are taking Enovid," he said, "our share of thrombophlebitis patients would be 710 cases. But we only have 26 reports of women taking Enovid who had been admitted to hospitals for the ailment."

According to Barbara Seaman, Searle was fudging the figures. In fact, she said, Searle's files were bulging with 132 reports from doctors whose patients had developed blood clots after taking oral contraceptives. Eleven of these women had died, but, Seaman wrote, no one at Searle seemed to take seriously a possible connection between The Pill and an increased risk of embolism. At the Chicago meeting, there was even "merriment about some of the deaths said to be associated with The Pill. One death, someone suggested, was caused by a 'tight girdle,' another by a 'long trip.' " The verbatim transcript, Seaman noted indignantly, showed "general laughter" at the joke.

## *Protecting The Pill*

G.D. Searle understood very well that the development of a successful contraceptive pill would be a major achievement in the pharmaceutical industry, "God's gift" to the company that got it to market first. "What they had in their laps," Paul Vaughn wrote in 1970, "was one of the classic golden eggs of the drug business, something in the great, money-spinning tradition of aspirin, penicillin, or purple hearts, but with advantages none of these possess. If the idea could be sold, the pill would have a virtually guaranteed sale to millions of women at the rate of 240 tablets a year throughout their child-bearing lives, from menarche to menopause with only such intervals as a woman chose in order to have a baby. [It was] a drug to be taken, for a perfectly valid reason, not by the sick, but by the healthy."

Certainly, the company had an enormous economic stake in protecting Enovid while it was being tested in Puerto Rico and afterward when it was released for sale in the United States. It did its job assiduously, refusing to acknowledge even the possibility of serious side effects.

But it would be a mistake to think that protecting its balance sheet was Searle's only motivation in defending The Pill. Like Planned Parenthood, Searle considered itself a partner in a noble quest to make a safe, effective, inexpensive birth control product widely available around the world. "I'm pretty sure that when history books are written," said Searle chairman John G. Searle in 1969, "our organization's greatest single contribution to mankind will be 'Enovid.' It is a positive answer to a world threatened by overpopulation, and the resulting poor subsistence, poor shelter and poor education that surplus people are forced to endure."

Searle and Planned Parenthood were hardly alone in their defense of The Pill. In fact, they were backed by an entire contraceptive establishment, a powerful network—mostly liberal, mostly white, mostly upper middle class—that drew strong financial support from members of the American industrial aristocracy and maintained strong natural ties to other white, upper-middle-class bastions of power with the ability to control health policy.

There was, for example, the American Society for the Control of Cancer, founded in 1913 and rechristened the American Cancer Society (ACS) in 1945. The ACS, which to this day does not include estrogens on its list of risk factors for breast cancer, was originally supported by "a few concerned citizens," including John D. Rockefeller, Jr., who became a major benefactor and whose own lawyer, Thomas Debevoise, served as the organization's secretary.* The American Cancer Society's all-male leadership was dominated in the early years by men from two other pillars of the medical community, the American College of Surgeons and the American Medical Association (AMA). On August 9, 1962, two days after FDA commissioner George Larrick forced G.D. Searle to warn U.S. physicians that taking Enovid might raise a woman's risk of blood clots, the AMA issued the following statement: "The American Medical Association has made a careful scientific review of oral contraceptives. The AMA found absolutely no evidence that the use of oral contraceptives [causes] thrombophlebitis (blood clots in a vein)."

The contraceptive research fraternity also seeded organizations such as the Rockefeller Institute (later Rockefeller

---

* In 1936, Rockefeller expanded the establishment's research and treatment capacities with a grant of $3 million and a million-dollar plot of land on the East Side of Manhattan for a new building at Memorial (later Memorial Sloan-Kettering) Cancer Center. In 1974, when New York governor Nelson Rockefeller's second wife, Happy, had double breast surgery there, the hospital was performing forty mastectomies every day.

University), the Population Council, and the Alan Guttmacher Institute, a statistical research unit created for Planned Parenthood in 1968 by Guttmacher when he retired as Planned Parenthood's president and later spun off as an independent organization.

As you would expect in any group of like-minded people, members moved easily from one point to another within this exclusive circle. For example, Elizabeth Connell, M.D., author of *The Menopause Book* (1977), served prominently on FDA advisory committees that certified to the safety of estrogens; she was also a member of the staff at the Rockefeller Foundation, spent time as chairman of the national medical committee of Planned Parenthood World Population, and served as an adviser or consultant to a number of pharmaceutical companies including some, such as Syntex, Ortho, and Searle, that made and sold birth control pills.

The establishment's influence extended into government (and therefore into health policy) through a series of two-way streets that included grants for contraceptive and cancer research as well as use of the American Cancer Society's multimillion-dollar fund-raising efforts and enormous army of volunteers (which one year numbered a full 1 percent of all the people in the country) as the "educational arm" of the federal government's National Cancer Institute (NCI).

All these people and organizations had a philosophical and intellectual stake in defending oral contraceptives. More important, they had the ear of the FDA, which, after Searle agreed in August 1962 to tell doctors about the increased risk of blood clots associated with The Pill, turned deaf to further arguments against oral contraceptives.

By early 1963, The Pill had been on sale just about two years. Despite the reports of side effects, it was the contraceptive of choice for more than a million American women.

The market for ERT was considerably smaller, estimated by one doctor at 6,000 to 12,000 women a year. But then, in February 1963, a fifty-two-year-old Brooklyn woman walked into a local gynecologist's office for a simple check-up and, just by showing up, set off the second American estrogen explosion.

# chapter 5

# Menopause Revisited 1963–1966

## *The Female Deficiency Disease*

In 1963, three years after the FDA approved the use of hormones as contraceptives, Robert A. Wilson, M.D., was an obstetrician-gynecologist in Brooklyn, New York, where he was on the staff of Methodist Hospital. Wilson believed that menopause was a deficiency disease. "By way of rough analogy," he wrote, "you might think of [it] as a condition similar to diabetes." He was certain it could be treated with female hormones, just as diabetes was treated with insulin, and in fact he had been doing just that for forty years, first with ovarian extracts, then with estrogen alone, and finally with estrogen plus progesterone.

Wilson decided how much estrogen an individual patient needed by scoring her performance on a "Femininity Index," a term he coined to describe the results of a microscopic examination of the cells in a sample of vaginal tissue.

The growth and maturation of cells in the lining of the vagina is influenced by estrogen. An adequate supply of estrogen assures that there will be enough mature cells in the vagina to make the vaginal walls supple and moist. At menopause, when estrogen secretion from the ovaries slows, the number of mature cells declines and the walls of the vagina become thinner and drier. According to Wilson's Index, if 80 percent or more of the cells in the vaginal smear were mature, a woman was producing sufficient amounts of estrogen; her body was "still feminine." A count of fewer than 80 percent mature cells was a "clear warning" that "femininity is waning," a condition Wilson contended could be remedied with estrogen replacement therapy (ERT).

When he talked about his work, Wilson sounded as romantic as a knight in shining armor who was, as he put it, saving women from "being condemned to witness the death of their own womanhood." Fittingly enough, the woman who was to make his name a household word arrived like an early Valentine's card, on February 13, 1963.

Despite her age, "Mrs. P.G." (Wilson's name for his famous patient) stood straight, her muscle tone was good, her breasts were firm, and her skin was "as smooth and pliant as a girl's." Even her neck was free of wrinkles. When Wilson asked whether she had been taking hormones after reaching menopause, Mrs. P.G. laughed and said she had not yet reached menopause. "I have never missed a period," she said. "I'm so regular astronomers could use me for timing the moon."

Wilson's first thought was that she was already taking post-menopausal hormone replacement therapy (HRT). He was wrong. A few days later, Mrs. P.G. called back to tell Wilson something she had forgotten to mention during her checkup: She was taking an estrogen/progestin birth control pill similar in composition to the regimen had Wilson been prescribing for menopausal discomfort. But Mrs. P.G. was not using it to relieve menopausal problems; she had started using the new pills for birth control in 1960 when she was forty-nine and simply never stopped.

Wilson found that fascinating. To date, he had been prescribing hormones only *after* women reached menopause and began to experience symptoms such as hot flushes. But here was Mrs. P.G., fifty-two years old, still menstruating, with no menopausal symptoms at all. Did that mean that if a woman started using hormones in the form of oral contraceptives and then continued to take The Pill for the rest of her life, she could avoid menopause?

To some extent, that depended on what exactly one meant by the phrase "avoiding menopause." Certainly, Wilson did not mean that women who used hormones would remain fertile and be able to conceive. While it is possible that at fifty-two Mrs. P.G. was still fertile because she had not yet entered menopause, it is equally possible that the periodic bleeding she called a menstrual period was actually the pseudo-menstrual, nonovulatory cycle experienced by women who follow an estrogen/progestin regimen for post-menopausal HRT.

More likely, Wilson's point was that women who used estrogen felt better and looked better. To find out if Mrs. P.G.'s birth-control-pill regimen would work as well for other women, Wilson set up a study with eighty-two patients, age thirty-two to fifty-seven. As he had hoped, twenty-six of the twenty-seven pre-menopausal women given birth control pills to "prevent menopause" never experienced hot flushes, dry skin, or thinning of the vaginal walls. The remaining fifty-five patients, who had already entered menopause, were given oral contraceptives to relieve existing symptoms. Fifty-one of them—93 percent—said taking hormones made their symptoms disappear.

From this small nonrandom sample in a study that ran less than two years, Wilson concluded that taking an estrogen/progestin oral contraceptive before menopause started could prevent symptoms from ever occurring, and taking The Pill after menopause started would relieve or totally eliminate any existing symptoms.

## *Publicizing ERT*

With these studies in hand, Wilson quickly became an "all-out advocate of hormone replacement therapy, preferably beginning as early as age 30."

"Women rich in estrogen," he said, "tend to have a certain mental vigor that gives them self-confidence, a sense of mastery over their destiny, the ability to think out problems effectively, resistance to mental and physical fatigue, and emotional self-control. Their emotional reactions are proportional to the occasion. They neither over-react hysterically, nor do they tend toward apathy. They are, as a rule, capable of facing the world with a healthful relaxed attitude and thereby to enjoy their daily life. They are seldom depressed. Irrational crying spells are virtually unknown among them. In a family situation, estrogen makes women adaptable, even tempered, and generally easy to live with. Consequently a woman's estrogen carries significance beyond her own well-being. It also contributes toward the happiness of her family and all those with whom she is in daily contact."

In 1966, Wilson published *Feminine Forever,* a book detailing his theories on estrogen replacement. The book sold more than 100,000 copies in its first seven months, and all through 1966, articles about the book and his own bylined pieces on estrogen therapy appeared in magazines as diverse as *New Republic, Time,* and *Vogue.*

A typical Wilson article appeared in the June 1966 issue of *Vogue.* The article listed therapeutic regimens for women in various age groups ranging from a sprightly seventeen to a dignified eighty-five. For the youngest ones, age seventeen to twenty-nine, whose estrogen deficiency might show up in their poor complexion; recurring acne; dull, lusterless hair; breasts that did not feel firm; or a tendency to gain weight after age twenty-five, Wilson proposed estrogen every day for the first three weeks of the menstrual cycle. For women age thirty to thirty-nine suffering from fat pads on hips and abdomen along with dry, sagging skin; dull hair; dry eyes and nasal passages; plus "loss of breast firmness," the prescription was daily estrogen for the first three weeks of the cycle, with progestins added the last two weeks if necessary. After age forty, virtually every woman would need some combination of estrogen and progesterone on a regular schedule for the rest of her life.

Wilson was reported to say that well past menopause a woman would need six-week cycles of daily estrogen with progestins added in the last ten days; when a woman withdrew from the progestins, she would experience bleeding, a kind of pseudo-menstrual period. He told *Look* magazine readers that feeling good and looking young weren't the only benefits of hormone therapy. Menopausal women who worried about accidental pregnancies would also be getting "automatic concurrent contraception as a *non-sought-after* and therefore theologically permissible *secondary* result. For millions of women with religious scruples, dependence on rhythm can be over at this period of their lives."

Many colleagues flocked to Wilson's campaign to make hormones standard therapy for post-menopausal women. Some even endorsed his hyperbolic claims. For example, in the introduction to *Feminine Forever,* Robert B. Greenblatt, chairman of the department of endocrinology at the Medical College of Georgia, wrote that "[Wilson] sounds the clarion call, awakening a slumbering profession to a woman's needs."

But others were put off by Wilson's single-mindedness, especially when they knew from their own experience that not all menopausal women actually required estrogen therapy. There were still serious doubts about the long-term effectiveness of hormones, and the authoritative *Medical Letter* even questioned whether estrogen replacement could really "preserve a youthful complexion or guard against heart attacks, dowager's hump or broken bones."

Eventually the media hype that had made Wilson's theories so popular brought him to the attention of the Food and Drug Administration, which began to look into how he conducted his research. Wilson treated his patients and ran his tests at the Wilson Research Foundation, an organization funded by, among others, Ayerst Laboratories, the manufacturers of the best-selling menopausal estrogen product, and G.D. Searle, developers and marketers of birth control pills. In addition to monetary grants, Searle had given Wilson supplies of Enovid to use in his studies of the effects of birth control pills on menopausal symptoms. But in November, the FDA told Searle that Wilson would no longer qualify as a Searle researcher on this subject because he was telling patients that Enovid was effective for menopausal discomfort even though no one had yet proven that to be true.

Neither had anyone shown that estrogens were safe. But one thing was certain: Although there had already been a few reports hinting at a higher incidence of endometrial cancer among women using post-menopausal ERT in 1966, the estrogen product causing the most trouble was neither ERT nor the DES prescribed for pregnant women. It was still The Pill.

# chapter 6

# An Inference of Blame 1966–1969

## Lawyers and Doctors

In 1966, when *Feminine Forever* was hitting the best-seller lists, the Food and Drug Administration issued its first *Report on the Oral Contraceptives*. Even though the agency had persuaded Searle to tell doctors about the possibility of blood clots for pill users, this new report said that there still wasn't enough information available either to confirm or refute a link between the drug and the condition.

Nonetheless, women continued to complain of pill-related discomfort; doctors continued to mail reports of pill-associated blood clots to the FDA; and soon enough, pill victims (or their survivors) started to call in the lawyers.

Raymond Black was one of those survivors. In May 1969, the thirty-five-year-old engineer from South Bend, Indiana, was in federal court in Des Moines seeking $750,000 in damages from Searle because in 1965 his twenty-nine-year-old wife, Elizabeth, had died from a pulmonary embolism while taking Enovid. Medical experts testifying for Black said that his wife's blood clot was triggered by the birth control pill, but Searle's medical witnesses countered with autopsy slides showing that Elizabeth Black had an infection of the heart muscle, which South Bend pathologist Chris A. Pascuzzi said made her "a perfect candidate for thrombosis of the vein." The jury sided with Searle but did ask the judge to tell the drug company to warn doctors and patients that oral contraceptives could be harmful. The judge, Robert Grant, made it clear that the request for a warning had no legal force.

If Searle prevailed in South Bend, it was a Pyrrhic victory. Within months, there were new lawsuits, including one in Buffalo, New York, where a couple filed a $1 million suit in federal court contending that a second Searle oral contraceptive, Ovulen, was responsible for the wife's developing various ailments, including blood clots in her lungs.

The reports of headaches, vision problems, and general malaise among other women using birth control pills continued apace, and there was a growing sense of unease about The Pill. Clearly, as pharmacologist Dr. Louis Lasagna of Johns Hopkins University Medical School told *The New York Times*, oral contraceptives were not "as harmless as water as some people have tried to lead us to believe."

Even so, in September 1969, an FDA Advisory Committee on Obstetrics and Gynecology released a 185-page *Second Report on Oral Contraceptives* concluding that, although about 255 of the 8.5 million women taking The Pill each year would die as a result of pill use, birth control pills were safe because their benefits still outweighed their risks.


## No Action from the FDA

The FDA's acceptance of those 255 deaths was particularly egregious in light of the results of a study the Advisory Committee had tucked right into its own presentation. The study, an analysis of data collected at forty-eight hospitals in Baltimore, New York City, Philadelphia, Pittsburgh, and

Washington, D.C., suggested that many (if not all) of the projected 255 deaths each year from The Pill might actually be preventable. It showed that women who took birth control pills were more than four times as likely to die of a blood clot than were women who used other forms of birth control. The study did not specifically designate estrogen as the cause of the blood clots, but Johns Hopkins University epidemiologist Philip E. Sartwell said there was an "inference" that the hormone was to blame.

The FDA Advisory Committee report also ignored the conclusions of the British Committee on Safety of Drugs, which in 1969 had again taken the lead by recommending that doctors no longer prescribe contraceptive pills containing more than 50 mcg (0.05 mg) estrogen. The FDA did advise doctors to prescribe the "low-dose" pills, but the agency did not get around to banning the use of birth control pills containing more than 50 mcg (0.05 mg) estrogen until 1988, a full eighteen years after the British threw them out. (When the new low-estrogen pill went on sale in Great Britain in April 1970, six months after the FDA report, English government researchers said it would reduce the incidence of blood clots among young British women by 25 percent and cut deaths from blood clots in half.)

But even if the low-estrogen pills produced fewer immediate side effects, they might still cause long-term damage such as cancers that would not show up for years. There was no way to tell because there simply were no long-term studies of estrogen replacement therapy. Nor could you look to the Puerto Rican trials of Enovid for guidance; the information wasn't there either.

The public perception, never discouraged by either the doctors who tested The Pill or G.D. Searle or the FDA, was that during the Puerto Rican trials several thousand women had taken oral contraceptives for at least a year. In fact, the researchers originally intended to follow no more than a hundred women. The constant turnover as women left the project and were replaced by others doubled the number of participants to 221 women who took the pill for more than two months. There were none who took it for longer than nine months.

When The Pill scientists said that they had compiled forty-seven "patient years" of experience with birth control pills in Puerto Rico, they meant simply that they had added up the total number of months the pill was used by each of the 221 women in the study and then divided by twelve. So the trials were useful for determining short-term side effects (although the reports of symptoms among women taking The Pill were disparaged as imaginary), but they were meaningless in any assessment of the risks of long-term pill use because nobody in the Puerto Rican trials used The Pill long term.

When it granted its initial approval for the sale of hormones as contraceptives, the FDA gave tacit recognition to the lack of knowledge regarding the safety of long-term use by limiting to two years the time any one doctor could prescribe The Pill for any one patient.

But there were no such limitations on the use of estrogen replacement therapy.

Even if there had been, that would not have addressed questions about the most frightening side effect of all: cancer.

# Definitions, Statistics, and Studies

# chapter 7

# Defining the Disease

## *What Is Cancer?*

C ancer isn't one disease; it is many. What they have in common is that all thrive by disrupting the normal growth and reproduction of body cells.

Ordinarily, our bodies produce cells characterized by one of three basic growth patterns. The first type of cell, known as "stem cells," have well-defined life cycles, such as the six-month life of a red blood cell. Stem cells reproduce and replace themselves as long as we are alive, which is why skin wounds heal so quickly and blood volume returns to normal relatively soon after we donate blood.

A second type of body cell is programmed to reproduce only a specific number of times. These cells are found in organs such as the kidney and the liver, as well as certain glands where there is theoretically no need for new growth once the body is mature and the organ or gland has grown to its "correct" size. That is why kidney or liver damage or failure constitutes a potentially life-threatening event. Finally, there is a third type of cell, one whose function is so specific and specialized that it does not regenerate at all. Nerves are made primarily of this kind of cell, and that is why nerve damage is usually permanent.

Cancer cells do not obey any of these rules. They continue to divide and reproduce without control. And unlike healthy cells, which do not implant themselves in "foreign" places, cancer cells invade surrounding tissue or spread via the lymphatic system or the bloodstream to establish beachheads in other parts of the body, a process known as metastasis. The aim of cancer treatment is to interrupt this process either by removing the cells from the body (surgery), destroying them where they hide (radiation), or interrupting their growth cycle so they cannot reproduce and spread (chemotherapy).

## *What Is Breast Cancer?*

Breast cancer is a malignant tumor that arises in the breast and may metastasize to other sites, usually lungs, bone, liver, and brain. Most breast cancers grow very slowly, causing no pain or symptoms until they are far advanced. Two exceptions are inflammatory breast cancer, which grows very quickly, turning the skin over the tumor red, warm, and painful, and Paget's disease, which sends its cells along ducts leading to the nipple and out onto the skin's surface where they produce a crusty eczemalike rash.

Until the introduction of mammography, breast cancer was almost always diagnosed late in the game, when the tumor, assumed to be a local phenomenon, had already established colonies throughout the body. As a result, surgery, no matter how radical, almost inevitably failed to cure the disease.

Today, mammography makes it possible to identify very early breast tumors, and a new armament of anticancer drugs enables oncologists to treat breast cancer as a systemic disease, attacking cells that have metastasized to distant sites throughout the body. Thus, for many women, breast cancer has been redefined from an imminently fatal disease to a chronic illness that (a) may never metastasize, or (b) may take so long to spread that the patient is likely to die of something else in the meantime.

But describing breast cancer solely in terms of its physical characteristics ignores its psychological impact on the victim.

Before the 1970s, a diagnosis of cancer was almost always a death sentence without appeal that doctors (and families) felt justified in hiding from the patient. As our understanding of the etiology and treatment of cancer has grown, however, some of the mystery and dread surrounding many forms of the disease has dissipated.

Today, we know that smoking causes lung cancer and may be implicated in a host of other malignancies such as cancer of the bladder, cancer of the esophagus, and cancer of the kidney. We know that prolonged exposure to sunlight raises the risk of skin cancer, that aflatoxins (food molds) raise the risk of stomach cancer, and that a high-fat, low-fiber diet may increase the risk of colon cancer. That means we can protect ourselves by not smoking, avoiding excess sunlight, protecting the food supply from spoiling (preservatives, it turns out, may actually prevent cancer), and consuming less fat and more fiber.

But there is no such simple way to reduce the risk of breast cancer, because no one has thus far been able to pinpoint with any degree of exactitude what causes the disease or which women are likely to develop it. As University of Cincinnati radiologist Myron Moskowitz told the National Conference on Breast Cancer in March 1988, 75 percent of all breast cancers occur in women with *no known risk factors*.* Finally, even though our doctors can find the tumors earlier, we do not yet have the long-term studies we need to find out

* A 1990 article in *Newsweek* put the no-risk-factor figure at 55 percent.

whether the new treatments applied to early tumors actually cure the disease or simply extend the time between diagnosis and death.

Sometimes it seems that all we can do is stare in horror at the numbers, which have more than tripled—from approximately 50,000 new cases in 1940 to more than 180,000 in 1992.

# Counting the Cases

## *Where the Numbers Come From*

Epidemiology is the science that tells you how common a disease is and how fast it is spreading. Epidemiological studies provide the simple, stark numbers that tell you how many new cases of a disease occur each year and how many people die of it. If analyzed correctly, they may also show a pattern that identifies the cause of a disease or explains why it is occurring in a certain population or during a specific period of time. For example, beginning in 1981, epidemiologists from the U.S. Centers for Disease Control (CDC) were able to link increasing reports of a previously rare cancer (Kaposi's sarcoma) to the appearance of a new disease, acquired immunodeficiency syndrome (AIDS), among gay men.

Before the turn of the century, however, epidemiology was a less sophisticated discipline. It focused mainly on counting the number of people suffering from contagious diseases such as tuberculosis or diphtheria. There were few attempts to find out either how many were getting cancer or how many were dying from it. Even so, starting early in the 1800s, it was possible to discern a steady increase in cancer mortality that climbed from about 20 cancer deaths for every 100,000

Americans in 1840 to 50 per 100,000 in 1880, on to 64 per 100,000 in 1900, the first year that formal statistics on cancer mortality in this country appeared in the U.S. Census.*

The mortality figures in the 1900 census came from certificates filed by doctors in a government-created Death Registration Area, ten states then accounting for about one-quarter of the national population. They showed cancers of all kinds accounting for 3.7 percent of the deaths in the United States, which made cancer the eighth leading cause of death, behind heart disease and stroke, influenza and pneumonia, tuberculosis, intestinal and stomach infections, "senility" and other ill-defined conditions of old age, kidney disease, and accidents.

In 1933 the government broadened its collection of mortality statistics to include death certificates from the entire country. The first statistics on cancer incidence appeared two years later, in 1935, when Connecticut established a Tumor Registry to collect information about the occurrence of specific cancers among people living in the Nutmeg State. These figures, from only one state, were used to predict national incidence when the fledgling National Cancer Institute (NCI) issued its first report in 1937.

The Connecticut Tumor Registry served as the basis for cancer incidence predictions until 1973, when NCI expanded its coverage by creating the Surveillance, Epidemiology and End Results (SEER) program.† SEER's mission was to make cancer statistics more accurate by broadening

---

* In epidemiological terms, *mortality* describes the total number of deaths per year; the *death rate* is the number of deaths in one year in a specific population such as every 100,000 American women. Likewise, the *incidence* of female breast cancer in America is the total number of new cases among American women in one year; the *incidence rate* is the number of cases in one year for a specific population, such as 100,000 American women or 100,000 American women younger than thirty-five.

† "End results" is a euphemism for "deaths."

the area from which they were collected, but the early SEER statistics were often criticized because the data were not collected at random and the population on which they were based was not varied enough to reflect all the races and ethnic groups living in the United States. For a long time, SEER data were limited to white people simply because the number of blacks, Hispanics, Asians, and other nonwhites in the SEER states and urban areas was too small to give a reliable estimate of risk for nonwhites and because the proportion of specific racial groups in the SEER areas did not accurately mirror their presence in the country as a whole.*

Today SEER gathers its numbers from areas that, taken all together, comprise about 10 percent of the population: Connecticut, Hawaii, Iowa, New Mexico, Utah, and the metropolitan areas of Atlanta, Detroit, San Francisco–Oakland, and Seattle–Puget Sound. The SEER population is still not perfectly representative of the country as a whole—for example, the racial composition of the SEER population does not accurately reflect the proportions of various non-white racial groups in the entire country—but careful monitoring has made the survey's incidence data more accurate.

Once SEER has compiled its incidence data, NCI and the National Center for Health Statistics (NCHS) of the U.S. Department of Health and Human Services use that information plus the information on mortality derived from

---

* For several years, this was one reason for challenging the validity of the early SEER statistics. To guarantee the accuracy of incidence rates, it is important that the population be varied and that it include people likely to be affected by the disease. For example, to track the incidence of breast cancer in the United States, you need a population that is overwhelmingly female (men, after all, account for only one case in 100) and includes a variety of ethnic groups. Some, such as Japanese-American women, appear to have a lower incidence of breast cancer than others, such as women of Jewish ancestry. Leaving out groups such as these may affect the results of a study.

death certificates across the country to draw up national cancer incidence statistics, statistics on death rates, and estimates of individual risk, such as the 1990 statement that an American woman's lifetime risk of breast cancer is 1-in-8.

The statistics produced by NCI and NCHS are intended primarily for use by health professionals. For the public at large, the best source of information on cancer incidence and mortality is *Cancer Facts and Figures,* an annual report issued by the American Cancer Society (ACS) that uses data from SEER and NCHS to predict how many new cases of cancer and how many cancer deaths will occur in the year ahead. These predictions from the ACS are the ones we are most likely to encounter in articles on cancer in consumer magazines, the numbers on which we base our impressions of cancer incidence and mortality.

## *Epidemiological Studies*

The SEER epidemiologists arrive at their mortality and incidence figures simply by adding up the numbers. To get more detailed information about any particular disease— that is, to identify the *cause* of the incidence or deaths—they rely on epidemiological studies. These studies generally fall into one of two categories, the cohort study (the name comes from the designation for a unit of a legion in the ancient Roman army) or the case/control study.

In a cohort study such as the trials of the birth control pill in Puerto Rico, an investigator picks a group of people (the cohort) and keeps detailed health records over a period of time to see what happens to them. The hope is that he or she will be able to identify the life-style or influences that cause (or prevent) specific health problems, or, as with The Pill trials, to see if a specific substance or product such as the birth control pill does what it is supposed to without causing unacceptable adverse effects.

In a case/control study, on the other hand, researchers compare "cases" (such as women with breast cancer) and "controls" (healthy women of similar age) to see what makes one group different from the other. Again, the hope is that finding the differences will provide a clue to what causes the disease.

Most cohort studies are prospective: They look forward, collecting data as they occur. Most case/control studies are retrospective: They look back in time, relying on other people's ability to keep accurate records or their subjects' ability to remember what happened. Given the likelihood that records will be less than perfect and the people will forget important details or gloss over unpleasant ones, retrospective studies are generally considered less reliable than prospective ones.

## *Confounding Factors*

To make sure that their numbers are correct, epidemiologists, including those at SEER, NCI, and ACS, must account for confounding factors, external influences that can change the meaning of statistics.

Suppose you want to test a new sleeping pill designed to help older people fall asleep fast and sleep soundly through the night. The scientific way to do it is to run a double-blind study in which you pick two groups of people, give one group the drug and the other group a placebo, but you do not tell either the subjects or the people running the test which group got what pill (hence the term *double-blind*). This reduces the chance that your subjects' reactions will be influenced by their own expectations or those of the people in charge of the test.

But for our purpose, which is to define the term *confounding factor,* a simpler system will do. This time, you pick five volunteers and tell them to take the pill at bedtime. The next morning, you ask them how they slept. Two of your volunteers tell you they fell asleep quickly and slept through the night like proverbial logs. The third volunteer says he fell asleep quickly but woke up often during the night. The last two say they didn't sleep a wink.

Assuming they are all telling the truth and that your new drug is responsible for their experience (two very big assumptions), your new drug worked for only two of your five volunteers, a 40 percent success rate, pretty poor for a new product meant to treat a very common problem.

When you dig a little deeper, though, you find that your happy sleepers went to bed at their usual time after a normal evening's dinner and activities, while your two sleepless volunteers, who usually go to bed around 11:00 P.M., actually took your pill very late at night after a heavy dinner accompanied by two drinks and two cups of caffeinated coffee.

All these things—staying up past a normal bedtime, eating a heavy meal late in the evening, consuming alcohol and caffeine late at night—can alter a person's normal sleep cycle. They are confounding factors that can change the results of your study.

---

**Age and breast cancer statistics.** As discussed above, the growing availability of mammography is one potential confounding factor for epidemiologists measuring the incidence of breast cancer in the United States. Another is the fact that our population is growing older.

Breast cancer is primarily a disease of older women, so it is logical to assume that with more women living longer, there will be more cases of breast cancer. But to find out for sure whether the steady increase in cases is due simply to the corresponding steady increase in the number of older women, epidemiologists "adjust" (or "standardize") their statistics to even out the effects of age. They do this by comparing the number of cases in the group they are studying, say the United States in 1990, to a "standard population," say the United States in 1950. The goal is to figure out how many cases of the disease would be considered normal if the proportion of people in each age group in 1990 were the same as the proportion of people in each age group in 1950.

For example, suppose that in 1950 there were only 100 women older than fifty in the United States and that in this population there were five cases of breast cancer, one for every twenty women older than fifty.

### Table 1. Age and the Incidence of Breast Cancer Among American Women, 1960–1990

| YEAR | WOMEN AGE 44+ (IN THOUSANDS) | BREAST CANCER CASES (TOTAL) | BREAST CANCER INCIDENCE PER 100,000 WOMEN | LIFETIME RISK | BREAST CANCER DEATHS (TOTAL) |
|---|---|---|---|---|---|
| 1960 | 26,169[1] | 63,000[2] | 72 | 1-in-14 | 23,970[2] |
| 1990– 1991 | 42,902[3] | 175,000[2] | 105+[2] | 1-in-9 | 44,500[2] |

[1] *Information Please Almanac 1960.* New York: McGraw-Hill, 1960, p. 525.
[2] Amerian Cancer Society.
[3] *World Almanac 1991.* New York: World Almanac, p. 555.
[4] Interview, Catherine Boring, American Cancer Society.

Now imagine that in 1990 there are 120 women older than fifty in the United States. If there are only six cases of breast cancer in this group, then the incidence of the disease has remained the same: one case for every twenty women.

But if there are now ten cases of breast cancer among these 120 older women, that would be one case for every *twelve* women.

In other words, it's not just the total number of cases that has gone up. The incidence rate (the number of cases for a specific group) has also risen, and clearly something other than the greater number of older women in the population is at work. (Death rates are corrected in the same way by the National Center for Health Statistics, which compares current death rates to the death rate for the population in the 1970 U.S. Census.)

# part three

# Hormones and Cancer

# chapter 9

# The Trail of Evidence 1961–1969

## *Contradictory Information*

In 1961, when The Pill went on sale in the United States, so few women, relatively speaking, had actually used estrogen at menopause or for menstrual disorders that there were only three studies, all retrospective, to document what happened to them. All three seemed to show that women using estrogen had a lower incidence of breast and reproductive cancers.

The early human studies of "long-term" estrogen use were flawed because they covered so few participants—only 618 women in all, some of whom had taken hormones for less than six months, far less than needed to find out if the hormone was carcinogenic.

How many people does it take to make a valid study? The short answer is "as many as possible." In practice, however, the number of people you need to produce reliable conclusions is generally determined by the natural incidence of the effect you want to study.

As a rule, the less common the effect, the more people you need to find it. For example, because breast cancer is relatively rare among young women, FDA epidemiologist Philip Corfman, M.D., once estimated that a one-year study designed to find out whether the use of oral contraceptives raises the risk of breast cancer in women twenty to forty years of age, would require 85,000 women. A similar one-year study to find out whether women who use oral contraceptives are more likely to give birth to malformed babies would require only 600 participants because birth defects in newborns are more common than breast cancers in young women. And, says Graham Colditz, M.D., of Harvard Medical School and Brigham and Women's Hospital, even these numbers may be too small to find an effect not immediately apparent.

Clearly the size of the early studies affected their accuracy. In addition, the data were muddied by the inclusion of pre-menopausal women (some as young as fifteen), and by the fact that some women had gotten androgens, not estrogens, while others got a combination of male and female sex hormones. As for the estrogen produced naturally in the body, its role in breast cancer was, to say the least, inconclusive. Pre-adolescent girls never developed breast cancer, which suggested that a woman's body needed some estrogen "priming" of the tissues to enable a tumor to take hold. Moreover, removing a woman's ovaries once she had breast cancer often slowed or reversed the course of the disease, which implied that if you did just the opposite, gave women estrogen as birth control pills or ERT, you might speed up the growth of any existing tumor.

The trouble was you couldn't generalize from these assumptions to say that high levels of estrogen caused breast cancer and low levels were protective; simple observation told you it wasn't always true. Breast cancer was *least common* (but potentially more dangerous) during pregnancy, when the natural production of estrogen soars, and *most common* after menopause, when the body's secretion of estrogen declines.

So, based on the existing studies, plus the limited experience with ERT and the Puerto Rican trials, doctors besieged by patients demanding the new antipregnancy pill found it entirely reasonable to assume that oral contraceptives would cause nothing more than the uncomfortable but nonfatal side effects experienced with ERT. Many even found it logical to hope that the extra hormones women got via oral contraceptives would be protective, a theory endorsed by estrogen enthusiast Robert Wilson.

In 1962 he published a report in the *Journal of the American Medical Association* detailing his experience prescribing estrogens over a twenty-seven-year period for at least 304 women age forty to seventy. Given the then-current incidence statistics, one could, by rights, expect to find eighteen reproductive cancers among these women. Dr. Wilson found none, and that led him to conclude that the evidence "indicates that estrogen and progesterone are prophylactic." As far as Wilson was concerned, female hormones didn't cause cancers of the breast; they prevented them.

But Wilson's assertions aside, there was no proof either way. This made a lot of people nervous, especially the epidemiologists, researchers, and physicians familiar with the studies of estrogen's effects on animals.

## Testing Drugs on Animals

When Cleopatra wanted to find out whether (and how fast) a new poison would kill an enemy, she tried it first on an unfortunate slave or prisoner, a no-nonsense testing method employed by monarchs through at least the seventeenth century. By the mid-1800s, however, the introduction of the scientific method, not to mention a slowly rising regard for the value of human life, led researchers to test their palliatives and remedies on animals instead of people.

Soon, the idea that anything that poisoned animals or made them sick would likely have the same effect on people was widely accepted. Miners carried caged canaries underground with them to detect the presence of invisible deadly gases, and Boston dentist William Morton tested his anesthesia on birds before trying it on people.

As cancer research matured, scientists also began to use animals to test a chemical's carcinogenicity. Some species were more susceptible than others to the effects of specific substances, but most experts agreed that anything causing cancer in a variety of laboratory mammals would probably cause cancer in people, too.* In fact, for several decades, the results of studies with a number of different species had consistently pointed to an unambiguous link between estrogen and cancer of the breast and reproductive organs.

In 1916, twenty years after Scottish surgeon Sir George Beatson demonstrated that removing a breast cancer patient's ovaries might slow the course of her disease, biologists A. F. C. Lathrop and L. Loeb published a report in the *Journal of Cancer Research* describing the same result in female mice. Edgar Allen and Edward Doisy's 1923 test to measure the effectiveness of ovarian extracts was based on the observation that injecting the ovarian material into female laboratory mice caused a sudden spurt in the growth of vaginal cells. Within a short time, scientists knew that this character-

---

* In the late 1950s, state-of-the-art biological technology carried this down the evolutionary scale when biochemist Bruce N. Ames of the Universiry of California, Berkeley, introduced a procedure that predicted a substance's carcinogenicity based on its ability to cause mutations in the structure of bacteria.

However, as Carl Djerassi pointed out in *The Politics of Contraception,* his 1979 history of birth control, the Ames test did not indict natural steroid hormones, and it was worthless in evaluating the nonsteroid synthetic estrogen DES because DES was toxic to bacteria. It killed them outright before anyone could tell whether there would be mutations.

istic, the ability to stimulate the rapid proliferation of body cells, was one measure of a chemical's potential carcinogenicity.

From 1932 through 1936, French biologist A. Lacassagne repeatedly produced tumors of the breast, uterus, testes, kidneys, bones, and other tissue in a variety of mammals by injecting the animals with large amounts of estrogens. In 1940 and 1941, American National Cancer Institute researchers Michael B. Shimkin and Hugh C. Grady showed that synthetic estrogens could also be hazardous. When Shimkin and Grady fed DES to their mice, either alone or in combination with the natural estrogen estrone, both the males and the females developed breast tumors. The tumors among the female mice were no surprise because the animals in the Shimkin-Grady tests, a strain known as C3H, had been bred especially for their sensitivity to breast cancer, and the females sometimes developed tumors spontaneously. But the males didn't—until they got the estrogens. Later, estone alone was used to induce breast tumors in laboratory rats.

In *Feminine Forever*, Robert Wilson dismissed biologist Lacassagne's studies during the 1930s as "ill-planned and misleading." The Shimkin-Grady tests cut no ice with researchers such as George and Olive Smith. The Smiths, who had promoted the use of DES for pregnant women in the belief that the extra estrogen would produce healthier babies, told Barbara Seaman twenty-six years later that "you can do all kinds of things to rats and mice by giving them overdoses."

But others found Lacassagne's work thoroughly reputable. Roy Hertz, the man who had tested Carl Djerassi's progestins at NIH in 1958, first on animals and then on human beings, and Edward F. Lewison, M.D., head of the breast cancer clinic at Johns Hopkins Hospital in Baltimore, repeatedly cited it in their own articles. Well into the 1980s, standard medical textbooks referred to it as proof that natural estrogens could cause cancer, at least in animals.

---

**A notable exception.** The only notable exceptions to this series of studies in which estrogens caused cancer in animals were six separate experiments with rhesus monkeys that ran between 1937 and 1950. In these six studies, none of the animals given estrogens developed overt cancers. No cancer of the breast. No cancer of the reproductive organs.

Because primates in general are so similar to human beings, and because rhesus monkeys in particular metabolize steroid hormones in a manner similar to human beings, it was tempting to give greater weight to these six studies than to all the others combined. In 1966, Robert Wilson said what a lot of people were thinking when he wrote that the "close relationship of monkey to man [means] these experiments are especially valid in evaluating estrogen in humans."

But there was another side to the story.

First, to run an animal study that will give you information you can reliably apply to human beings, you have to include enough animals so that you eliminate the possibility that your results occurred by chance. The six monkey studies used a total of only twenty-five different animals.

As Carl Djerassi said, an animal's life span is different from that of a human being, and these tests did not run long enough to approximate the length of time a woman might be using estrogens. In 1960 an American woman had an average life expectancy of about seventy-three years. If she reached menopause at an average age of fifty and followed Robert Wilson's advice, she might expect to be using estrogen replacement therapy for more than twenty years. As for birth control pills, while the FDA had put a limit of two years on prescriptions when it approved Enovid, if the pills turned out to be safe as well as effective, a woman might be using them for as long as thirty years. Because monkeys have an average life expectancy of fifteen years, the test would have to run for six and a half years to equal the thirty years a woman might be using estrogen birth control pills. Only four of the twenty-five monkeys in the six estrogen studies got hormones for four years or longer.

But the worst aspect of the primate studies was not that they used too few animals for too short a time. It was that the results were misrepresented. Contrary to what the hormone advocates said, the monkey studies *did not* exonerate estrogen. As Roy Hertz wrote in 1967, although none of the animals developed full-blown cancers, in at least two of the studies, one in 1935 and one in 1950, estrogen injections caused pre-cancerous changes in the cells of the cervix and endometrium. Like all the animal tests before them, these six studies confirmed the fact that estrogen was a potential carcinogen. In May 1969 the ACS and the Cancer Control Program of the U.S. Public Health Services sponsored the First National Conference on Breast Cancer in Washington, D.C. At the conference Harvard researchers Brian MacMahon and Philip Cole said that based on studies in which ovariectomy had reduced the risk of breast cancer in rodents, cats, dogs, and women, and treatment with estrogen had induced breast cancers in laboratory animals, the "indirect evidence" of estrogen's ability to cause cancer was "overwhelming."

Why, you may be wondering, wasn't all this taken as a signal to at least go slow on estrogens for women?

The answer is simple. In 1969, our drug tests were still focused on immediate adverse effects, such as the blood clots triggered by The Pill, not long-term ones such as reproductive cancers. When laboratory animals were given estrogens, they developed reproductive tumors within a fairly short time. That did not happen to women using DES, The Pill, or

ERT. The drugs worked. Women taking DES delivered healthy babies; women taking birth control pills did not become pregnant; women taking ERT were spared the discomforts of menopause.

At the same time, however, the incidence of breast cancer was still edging up. In 1960, the lifetime risk was 1-in-14. Now, at the end of the decade, it was 1-in-13. And no one could tell you why.

# chapter 10

# Marking Time 1969–1971

## *Doubts and Warnings*

In the two-year period from 1969 to 1971, the American Cancer Society sponsored two major conferences on breast cancer, and the U.S. Senate held a series of full-dress hearings on the safety of oral contraceptives. But the appearance of activity was misleading. In reality, the scientific airplanes were circling in the air, waiting for someone—or some study—to tell them where to land.

One prominent critic of unrestricted estrogen therapy was the National Institutes of Health's Roy Hertz. Once the pill was actually on the market as an estrogen/progestin combination rather than the progestin-only product he had tested, Hertz began to worry about its long-term safety, particularly in regard to breast cancer. By 1963, when he was chief of the endocrinology branch of NCI, Hertz had come to believe that doctors should avoid any unnecessary treatment with hormones because of the possibility that estrogens might cause cancer. At a symposium in New York jointly sponsored by the New York Academy of Sciences, the American Cancer Society, and the National Cancer Institute, Hertz argued against the use of hormones as a long-term means of birth control.

Four years later, as professor of obstetrics and gynecology at George Washington University, Hertz dismissed the idea that one could predict that birth control pills were safe based on the fact that there were only a few reports specifically linking ERT to reproductive cancers. "These generalizations," he warned, "ignore some serious limitations in our epidemiologic knowledge over the past 25 years. Past clinical experience relates almost entirely to the use of estrogens for the control of symptoms in women of menopausal or post-menopausal age. In addition, a very limited number of young women suffering from artificially induced menopause, ovarian insufficiency, menstrual disorders, and other gynecologic problems have also been treated . . . [and] it is not valid to equate a past experience in predominantly older patients with what should be anticipated in younger women particularly with respect to breast cancer."

In 1969, at the First National Conference on Breast Cancer in Washington, where Harvard epidemiologists Brian MacMahon and Philip Cole had pointed to the indirect evidence linking estrogen to reproductive cancers in animals, Hertz meticulously detailed the case against the widespread, indiscriminate use of estrogens.

Look, he said in effect, what we have here is a substance, estrogen, known to stimulate the growth of existing metastatic cancers. Just because nobody has yet been able to document an upsurge of breast cancers among women who used birth control pills or post-menopausal estrogens doesn't mean the drugs are safe. After all, it takes a long time, sometimes decades, for cancers to show up in people who have been exposed to such known carcinogens as X-rays, benzene, coal tar, soot, and radioactive paints and ores.

What's more, he argued, it was reasonable to consider that what people knew about estrogen and breast cancer in 1969 was analogous to what they had known about cigarettes and lung cancer before epidemiological studies zeroed in on smoking as the primary cause of lung cancer. As far as estrogens and cancer were concerned, the likelihood was that worse was yet to come, perhaps sooner than anyone expected. "Although the peak incidence of carcinogenic responses may be expected to follow a full decade," Hertz warned, "one would expect a substantial scatter of cases a few years before this peak, and we are currently approaching this period in the course of events for substantial numbers of women."

Saying all this put Hertz in the apparent minority, but he was not without influential supporters. "In my opinion," said NCI epidemiologist John C. Bailar III, in a review of the papers presented at the conference, "there is no sound basis for assuring any woman that any dose, of any estrogen, given for any reason, is safe."

## *The Nelson Hearings*

On Wednesday, January 14, 1970, nine years and eight months after the FDA approved the use of hormones for birth control, the U.S. Senate became a player in the continuing drama of The Pill. Responding to the chorus of complaints about birth control pills ranging from the first reports of blood clots in 1961–1962 to Raymond Black's $750,000 lawsuit against Searle, Senator Gaylord Nelson (D-Wisconsin), chairman of the Senate Subcommittee on Monopoly of the Select Committee on Small Business, convened a Senate panel to inquire into the safety of oral contraceptives.

Anyone who walked into the Nelson hearings without checking the calendar could be forgiven for thinking he had stumbled into a rerun of the 1960s. The decade had changed but the arguments were the same.

On January 15, Roy Hertz showed up to warn that the pill was still experimental. There were, he said, only two things about oral contraceptives that had been substantiated beyond a reasonable doubt: They prevented conception and caused blood clots. As for the possibility that they might also be carcinogenic, he told the senators that estrogens were "to cancer what fertilizer is to the wheat crop."

Following Hertz, a steady stream of doctors and scientists came forward to warn that oral contraceptives might cause cancer, damage genes, or harm the children of women who took birth control pills by accident without knowing they were pregnant. But these charges were surmises based on extrapolations from animal studies or from an individual researcher's understanding of human reproductive physiology. There were still no conclusive human studies to prove them right. So it was no surprise that on January 17, the American College of Obstetricians and Gynecologists issued a statement deploring "inaccurate or sensational reports" about The Pill.

The Nelson hearings were big news on the front pages of newspapers across the country, and so was the poll released by the Gallup organization on February 1, 1970. According to Gallup, 18 percent of the American women using oral contraceptives had recently switched to another form of birth control, and another 23 percent were seriously thinking about doing the same thing. Gallup said that many of these women made their decision based on the previously cited warnings issued by experts testifying at the Nelson hearings, the kind of statement that prompted gynecologist Elizabeth Connell of Emory University to complain that the publicity generated by the hearings was causing panic among pill users that would, she warned, produce "dozens of unwanted pregnancies."

In March, after the Nelson panel disbanded with 1,402 pages filling three volumes of testimony, the FDA, under threat of a lawsuit from the American College of Obstetricians and Gynecologists and the newly created National Women's Health Network, finally drafted a new package insert for birth control pills. It warned, at last, that using oral contraceptives might increase a woman's risk of blood clots and stroke.

There was no warning about cancer. But you could feel the first faint tremors of an official unease later in the year. Reacting to the hearings, the Council on Drugs of the American Medical Association issued a statement saying that even though there wasn't enough information to come to a definite conclusion about whether oral contraceptives caused breast and reproductive cancers in human beings, the possibility that oral contraceptives might stimulate the growth of some existing tumors of the breast and ovary could not be ignored. "Patients should be carefully examined periodically," the Council concluded, "and those who have or have had a known or suspected hormone-dependent tumor should not use this method of contraception."

---

**New rules, new dissent.**   Back in 1962, after the thalidomide scandal in which one lone FDA scientist, Dr. Frances Kelsey, defied her superiors and went public with her fight to keep off the American market a sedative known to cause serious birth defects, the FDA had revised its drug approval process to require, among other things, that all new drugs be proven safe and effective in animals before they could be used for human beings.

Now, in 1972, two years after the Nelson hearings, the FDA created a special set of rules for testing contraceptive drugs. Henceforth, manufacturers would have to test these drugs for two years in rats, dogs, and monkeys before moving on to human trials. While the human trials were under way, the manufacturers would have to continue their canine studies for seven years and their monkey studies for ten, time periods considered reasonable for the assessment of long-term risks.

Reacting to this new stringency, a panel of scientists from the World Health Organization (WHO) said that applying data from experimental animals was misleading, because "it is impossible to assess the comparability of dosage and life spans." Pill developer Carl Djerassi had also sounded the same caution, writing that "because of the enormous diversity in the reproductive processes of animal species and the widely divergent effects of steroid sex hormones on different species, it is exceptionally difficult to extrapolate to humans data from administering steroid drugs to experimental animals."

It was a point well taken. Female dogs, for example, are much more likely than women to develop breast cancer and might be exquisitely more sensitive than women to estrogen stimulation. But in the main, the reproductive community embraced the idea of animal tests, which were valuable in predicting a chemical's ability to cause birth defects as well as cancer.

## *False Reassurances*

When a regulatory arm of the federal government, such as the SEC or the FDA, reaches an agreement with someone who has broken its rules, the offender generally signs a document called a Consent Decree. In principle, signing means that the offender denies having violated the law in the past and promises not to do so in the future, a statement ordinary people usually translate as, "I didn't do it, and I'll never do it again."

That, in a nutshell, was the medical establishment's argument about estrogen and breast cancer in 1971.

At the beginning of the year, the American Cancer Society estimated that there would be 70,000 new cases of breast cancer in the United States and 31,000 deaths. At the end of April, there was an unsettling article in the *New England Journal of Medicine* (*NEJM*): Three physicians at Harvard School of Medicine reported the discovery of a rare form of vaginal cancer diagnosed in seven young women aged fifteen to twenty-two who had been born between 1946 and 1951 to women who had used DES while pregnant.

It was the first real evidence that estrogens might cause cancer in human beings, although the cancer did not occur in the person who took the drug. The *NEJM* editorial called for a central clearinghouse to track similar cases of vaginal disease, but one month later, on May 17, when the ACS's Second National Conference on Breast Cancer convened at the Century Plaza Hotel in Los Angeles, the big news was the lack of a connection between hormones and breast cancer. As the headline on the "Special to *The New York Times*" story from the Los Angeles conference read: "Study Finds No Evidence That Breast Cancer Is Linked to Pill."

The study's author was Oxford University epidemiologist Martin Vessey, who had interviewed 436 women at five different hospitals in London. Half the women were hospitalized for breast cancer or benign breast disease; the other half for unrelated conditions. Each was asked what method of birth control she had been using, and although Vessey himself admitted that the answers made for "statistically uncertain" data—as with all retrospective studies, it was hard to be sure that the women were remembering things right—he nonetheless considered the information "very reassuring" because there did not seem to be any apparent relationship between a woman's choice of birth control and her risk of developing breast disease.

At the Los Angeles gathering, this appraisal was endorsed by epidemiologist Philip E. Sartwell of Johns Hopkins, who had come to a similar conclusion based on his own continuing study of more than 800 women at Johns Hopkins Hospital in Maryland. Like the British researchers, Sartwell, who in 1969 had called estrogen the likeliest cause of the blood clots suffered by women using birth control pills, found no evidence of an increased risk of breast cancer among women using female hormones.

But Vessey and Sartwell's two studies did not convince Roy Hertz, who called the data superficial. "You need at least 10 years of follow-up to detect a relationship," he told Jane E. Brody of *The New York Times,* "and most women have not used the pill that long."

Once again, the man who had been the first to test Carl Djerassi's progestins on human beings had a philosophical ally in Edward Lewison. A practicing physician and the head of the breast cancer clinic at Johns Hopkins, Lewison felt a responsibility to real patients who might be at real risk. Given what he described as the "well-known" fact that even small doses of estrogens could stimulate the growth of existing cancers, Lewison called on the men and women attending the conference to think about the ominous possibility that a woman's long-term use of estrogens for ERT or birth control might stimulate a small undiagnosed cancer or carcinoma-in-situ over the line into invasive malignancy.

"There has always been a great deal of controversy regarding the relationship of estrogen to breast cancer," says Lewison, who retired from Johns Hopkins in 1988. "But based on my own experience in my practice and many various epidemiologic studies, I felt that my position was right. I am still on the fence about estrogens, because there have been cases in my practice where I believe it either aggravated a small, incipient breast cancer or promoted a new one."

Lewison agreed with the cautionary statement the AMA Council on Drugs had issued in 1970. In fact, he had put together his own list of the women who might be at risk from oral contraceptives and probably should avoid all estrogens entirely:

1. Women with a strong family history of cancer
2. Women with a history of cancer of one breast
3. Women with recurrent chronic cystic mastitis
4. Women with currently noninvasive breast tumors (carcinomas-in-situ)
5. Women who had an "abnormal" mammogram*

As for the rest of the women taking estrogen, those who were not in one of these high-risk groups, there was no short-cut, quick-and-easy way to find out what their chance might be of ending up with cancer.

They, Lewison said, would simply have to wait for "the tyrant of time" to deliver his "final reckoning of the risks."

---

* Today, Lewison says he would add "the presence of genetic bio-markers."

# chapter 11

# First Reckoning 1975

## The Right Questions

In November 1971, the Food and Drug Administration issued a bulletin warning physicians against prescribing DES for pregnant women, yet sales continued to climb. Soon the antimiscarriage pill was being promoted as a "morning after" pill that could keep a fertilized egg from implanting in the womb. Birth control pills and estrogen replacement therapy also remained popular with about 8.5 million women on The Pill and another 2 million using hormones to ease their passage through menopause.

But now, driven by the need for an answer to the questions posed by people such as Lewison and Hertz, the number of studies looking for a link between estrogen and breast cancer began to grow. For the first time, rather than waiting for a trend to develop, epidemiologists began to aggressively seek solutions to the puzzle of the hormone's relationship with the disease.

The first question on everyone's list was still whether estrogen could be linked directly and conclusively to reproductive cancers among women on ERT or birth control pills.

If the answer turned out to be yes, then the next question was how a woman's age affected her susceptibility. Women using ERT had suffered only minor discomfort; women using birth control pills had developed immediate, sometimes life-threatening side effects. Would the same balance—negligible effects for older women, serious problems for the young—hold for estrogen and cancer?

Was a high dose of estrogen more hazardous than a low dose? Was short-term use safer than long-term use, or was the length of use irrelevant to estrogen's ability to cause malignant change in body tissue? Finally, what about the other known or suspected risk factors for breast cancer, such as the presence of benign breast disease, the number of children a woman had delivered, and her family history of breast cancer? Did estrogens in The Pill or ERT act independently of these risk factors, or was the combination synergistic?

For four years after the ACS's Second National Conference on Breast Cancer, these questions hung in the air unanswered.

Then in the fall of 1975, Edward Lewison's allegorical "tyrant of time" delivered its first irrefutable answers to questions about a direct link between estrogen therapy and human cancers. Between October 1, 1975, and August 16, 1976, six new reports were published, each one tying the use of an estrogen product to a directly increased risk of cancer of the female reproductive organs. The first (from San Francisco) and the last (from Kentucky) linked estrogens to breast cancer. We will see them later. It is the four in between, linking estrogens to cancer of the uterus, that interest us now.


## Estrogen and Endometrial Cancer: Bad News from the West Coast

Even before estrogen was isolated and identified in 1929, scientists knew that something, a mysterious "female principle" in ovarian tissue, triggered a rapid proliferation of cells in the reproductive organs of female laboratory animals. By 1945 they knew that this kind of unregulated cell growth might be a prelude to cancer. Two years later, cancer researcher Saul Gusberg, M.D., published a report in the December 1947 issue of the *American Journal of Obstetrics and Gynecology* suggesting that the "promiscuous" use of post-menopausal estrogen replacement therapy might be to blame for a reported increase in cases of uterine bleeding among post-menopausal women suffering from pre-malignant changes in the lining of the uterus.

Gusberg's warning may have played a part in temporarily slowing the spread of ERT, but with the 1966 publication of *Forever Female,* the prescription of ERT surged forward once again.

Now the results of this widespread use of post-menopausal hormones were emerging for all to see.

On October 31, 1975, Donald F. Austin, M.D., M.P.H., director of the California Tumor Registry, announced that the number of cases of cancer of the uterus in the San Francisco Bay area had jumped 50 percent between 1969 and 1973. And the same thing was happening elsewhere in the country. Some observers suggested that it might be caused by an increase in early detection or a trend to a diet higher in animal fats, but Austin brushed these ideas aside. Because the increase was most apparent among affluent white women over fifty, the women most likely to be using estrogens to relieve menopausal symptoms, he blamed it squarely on the growing use of female hormones for the treatment of menopausal distress.

The next month, in the November 1975 issue of *Obstetrics and Gynecology,* Steven Silverberg, M.D., and Edgar L. Makowski, M.D., of the University of Colorado School of Medicine switched targets, this time taking aim at oral contraceptives. Reading through the records of the "Registry for Endometrial Carcinoma in Young Women Taking Oral

Contraceptives," they had discovered a curious fact. Among the twenty-seven young women age twenty-one to thirty who had developed endometrial cancer, every one whose cancer had developed silently, without such warning signs as abnormal uterine bleeding or cystic ovaries, had been using a form of oral contraceptives known as "sequentials."

At the time, sequential birth control pills selling under brand names such as Oracon, Ortho-Novum SQ, and Norquen, accounted for about 10 percent of all the oral contraceptives sold in the United States. Unlike the estrogen/progestin combination, which delivered both hormones together in a single pill, the sequentials dispensed them separately on a schedule similar to what a woman might experience during a natural menstrual cycle in which estrogen predominates during the first half and progesterone at the end.

Women using sequential pills took estrogen alone for fifteen to sixteen days, followed by five to six days of combined estrogen and progestin, followed by seven days with no pills at all. As a result, they went through a relatively long period of unopposed estrogen stimulation—the fifteen or sixteen days of estrogen alone plus a week of a low dose of endogenous estrogen—during which the growth of the lining of the uterus continued unchecked by progestins. Silverberg and Makowski thought this might be the cause of an increase in the number of cases of endometrial cancer among young women. But the link between sequential pills and a higher risk of endometrial cancer was never proven.*

---

* Nevertheless, an FDA Advisory Committee soon recommended a new label for the sequentials warning that they were not as safe and effective as the combination pills. On February 25, 1976, Mead-Johnson, Ortho Pharmaceuticals, and Syntex Labs, the three major drug companies marketing the sequential pills, announced that they were withdrawing their products from the market because of "new evidence" tying the pills to endometrial cancer.

The ink was hardly dry on that page before the December 4 issue of the *New England Journal of Medicine* came out with not one but two new reports connecting post-menopausal estrogens to endometrial cancer.

Once again, the bad news was coming from the West Coast. Researchers at the Kaiser-Permanente Medical Center in Los Angeles and the University of Washington in Seattle had found a dramatic rise in the incidence of uterine cancer.* As in San Francisco, the increase was occurring among older women using estrogen replacement therapy. Therefore, there was no doubt that the hormone was involved. More important, where Austin, Silverberg, and Makowski had simply noted an increase in the number of cases, now epidemiologists began to quantify the estrogen-related increase in individual risk as well.

## Calculating Individual Risk

When an epidemiologist talks about risk, he or she means the possibility that one person, such as an American woman, will experience a specific effect, such as cancer. A good example of this kind of risk prediction is the National Cancer Institute's 1992 estimate that an American woman's lifetime risk of breast cancer is currently 1-in-8.

A second epidemiological term, relative risk, measures the risk experienced by members of a specific group, such as women using ERT, against a "norm" set by another group, such as women who do not take estrogen.

---

* The Kaiser-Permanente Medical Care Program is the oldest and largest of the nation's health maintenance organizations (HMOs). Founded in 1938 by industrialist Henry Kaiser, it now serves nearly 7 million patients, employs more than 9,000 physicians, and operates medical centers and hospitals in sixteen states and the District of Columbia.

The norm is expressed by the number 1.0. If you think of 1.0 as shorthand for 100 percent, you can see that a relative risk of 0.9 is 10 percent lower than normal, while a relative risk of 1.9 is 90 percent higher than normal.

Another way to express relative risk is to describe it as a multiple of the normal risk. For example, a relative risk of 1.9 is a risk "1.9 times normal" or "nearly double the normal risk."

In 1975, an American woman who was past menopause, had not had a hysterectomy, and was not taking estrogens had about one chance in 2,000 each year of developing endometrial cancer. Which was why the epidemiological community sat up and took notice at the beginning of November when Harry K. Ziel, M.D., and William D. Finkle, Ph.D., unveiled the results of an analysis of the records of women enrolled in the Kaiser-Permanente Health Plan in Los Angeles.

According to Ziel and Finkle, when a post-menopausal woman starting using ERT, her annual risk of endometrial cancer soared to 1-in-250, eight times higher than the norm. Women who used estrogens for no longer than five years had a slightly lower risk, just about five times higher than the risk for nonusers; women who stuck with ERT for seven years or more had a risk nearly fourteen times that of women who had never used estrogens at all.

Ziel and Finkle's frightening numbers were supported by a second article in the same issue of the *Journal,* a University of Washington case/control study comparing 117 endometrial cancer patients with women suffering from other forms of cancer. The statistics compiled by Donald C. Smith, M.D., were less dramatic but equally alarming. In Smith's study, women using post-menopausal hormones were, on average, 4.5 times more likely than nonusers to develop endometrial cancers.

Like G.D. Searle, which in 1962 had failed to warn doctors and patients that taking birth control pills might raise a woman's risk of blood clots, Ayerst Laboratories, the makers of Premarin (the best-selling post-menopausal estrogen product), denied any connection between ERT and endometrial cancer. In a "Dear Doctor" letter denounced by FDA commissioner Alexander Schmidt as "misleading and irresponsible," Ayerst told the nation's physicians that the "weak" studies did not demonstrate a link between estrogen and cancer of the uterus.

But Ayerst's defense did not wash. The West Coast studies were just too compelling. For a few years the case seemed settled: Estrogen was a clear risk factor for endometrial cancer.

Then something strange happened: A study appeared showing that in young women exactly the opposite was true.

## Younger Women, Lower Risk

In October 1980, researchers at the Kaiser-Permanente Medical Center in Walnut Creek, California, released to the press advance information regarding a report to be published in the December issue of the *Journal of Reproductive Medicine*. The Kaiser-Permanente project was a prospective cohort study established in 1967 to identify the causes of death and major forms of disease among 16,638 women from suburban communities around San Francisco who were enrolled in the Medical Care Program at the Walnut Creek center. By 1977 the investigators had been following their subjects for ten years. What they found when they sat down to analyze a decade's worth of information was a significantly lower incidence of fibrocystic breast disease, "strong" protection against endometrial cancer, and "weak" protection against ovarian cancer among young women using birth control pills.

In other words, although ERT appeared to raise the risk of endometrial cancer in older women, estrogen/progestin oral contraceptives might actually lower the risk for young women.

Could this be true?

The possibility that it was grew stronger two weeks later when the *New England Journal of Medicine* published the results of an analysis by Boston University epidemiologist David W. Kaufman and a team of researchers from eight different hospitals and universities that showed pretty much the same results. In the Northeast, as in California, women using birth control pills had a lower-than-expected rate of cancers of the uterus. Women who took The Pill for at least a year had only half as many endometrial cancers as nonusers. After three years, a woman using oral contraceptives was 66 percent less likely than a woman using some other kind of birth control to develop endometrial cancer, and the protection conferred by The Pill seemed to last for as long as five years after she stopped taking it.

Since 1980, these two patterns—a lower risk of endometrial and ovarian cancer for young women using birth control pills versus a higher risk of endometrial cancer for post-menopausal women using ERT—have been firmly supported by a wealth of epidemiological data.

By 1991 a comparison of six different studies of the relationship between oral contraceptives and reproductive cancers showed that using The Pill for one year lowered a woman's risk of ovarian cancer by 20 percent. After two years, the risk was 40 percent below normal; after four years, 60 percent. A similar article the same year in the medical journal *Contraception,* which compared fifteen studies on The Pill and cancer of the ovary, came to the same conclusion. In thirteen of the fifteen studies, women using birth control pills were from 20 percent to 70 percent less likely than other women to develop ovarian cancer, and in the fall of 1992, Ortho Pharmaceutical Corporation produced the first consumer advertisement claiming health benefits for The Pill. "There is evidence," the FDA-approved copy read, "that Pills such as Ortho-Novum 7/7/7 may provide some protection against developing ovarian cancer and cancer of the lining of the uterus."

As for the cause-and-effect relationship between estrogens and endometrial cancer among older women, that, too, has been confirmed by follow-up studies.

In 1991, one well-known standard medical textbook, *Harrison's Principles of Internal Medicine*, estimated that women using post-menopausal estrogens were 500 to 700 percent more likely than nonusers to develop endometrial cancer, and some experts now suggest that ERT may be responsible for an average of four to eight extra cases of endometrial cancer a year for every 1,000 women with intact uteruses who are using the hormones.*

At the end, sorting out the different roles estrogens might play in the development of uterine and ovarian cancer had been relatively easy. Nobody could say that about the search for a connection between estrogens and breast cancer.

---

* Because they assume this to be caused by unopposed estrogen stimulation of the lining of the uterus, which triggers a pre-cancerous proliferation of endometrial tissue (endometrial hyperplasia), most American physicians now prescribe progestins along with estrogens for post-menopausal women who have not had a hysterectomy. Women who take both hormones often experience cyclic bleeding that resembles a menstrual period because, like natural progesterone, which tells the uterus to shed its thickened lining if an egg released at ovulation is not fertilized and implanted in the uterus, progestins also cause the estrogen-thickened uterine lining to slough away. To date, the epidemiological evidence strongly suggests that the estrogen-progestin regime is less likely than estrogen alone to cause endometrial cancer.

For at least seventy years, most animal studies had shown a distinct relationship between the administration of estrogen and the development of breast tumors. But there were no data to show a similar relationship in women. One study in print linked estrogens to breast cancer, but it applied to men, not women: In 1968, the *British Medical Journal* published a report documenting breast cancer deaths among men who took estrogen after undergoing sex-change operations.

But then, in October 1975, the very same month in which the first studies linking estrogen to an increased risk of endometrial cancer among women using ERT were published, there finally appeared a study linking use of birth control pills to an increased risk of breast cancer.

Once again, the bad news was coming from the West Coast.

# The Pill and Breast Cancer

# chapter 12

# An Important Warning 1970–1975

## An Obvious Question

For thirty years, from 1940 to 1970, the incidence of breast cancer among American women had continued to rise in every age bracket from twenty through eighty-five, in some instances by as much as 60 percent.

By 1970 there were 25,000 breast cancer deaths a year. Every day in the United States, sixty-eight women died of the disease.

Finding the connection between estrogen replacement therapy and endometrial cancer had stimulated the search for a similar relationship between estrogens and breast cancer. The epidemiologists looking for a link to ERT were working parallel to those looking for a link to The Pill, but for clarity's sake, it is easier to follow first what happened with The Pill and then turn to what happened with ERT.

The story of The Pill and breast cancer begins in earnest in 1970 in California where Ralph Paffenbarger was looking for a solution to the mystery of the rising breast cancer rates.

Paffenbarger had trained to be a pediatrician, but he never practiced as one. Instead, he carved out a career as an epidemiologist specializing in infectious and chronic diseases at the National Institutes of Health (NIH) in Washington, D.C. His special interest was poliomyelitis; when the introduction of the Salk vaccine put an end to the annual terror of the polio epidemics, he retired from NIH and, like so many other Americans, headed for California. Once there, he joined the California State Department of Health's Bureau of Chronic Diseases.

Today, Paffenbarger, who is professor of epidemiology at Stanford University School of Medicine, recalls that by 1970, "we had done studies on heart disease and cancer, and breast cancer was clearly one of the more important cancers. We were looking for new things that might explain the rising incidence. Was The Pill involved? It was an obvious question and we just naturally fell into it."

Paffenbarger joined forces with Elfriede Fasal, M.D., an obstetrician/gynecologist and epidemiologist at the State Department of Health. Together, they set up a case/control project designed to track what effect (if any) using birth control pills had on the risk of breast cancer and/or benign breast diseases such as chronic cystic mastitis among women admitted to nineteen San Francisco Bay–area hospitals between January 1, 1970, and December 31, 1972.

After leaving the hospital, each woman in the study was interviewed by a nurse who asked detailed questions about her choice of birth control, her menstrual history, her pregnancies, her use of hormones, and her general medical condition, paying special attention to breast disease and disorders of the reproductive organs. Any discrepancies or inconsistencies were to be resolved by consulting the woman's doctor or her hospital records.

Nearly three years went by as Paffenbarger and Fasal analyzed the mountain of material from these interviews. In the interim, America's view of breast cancer underwent a sea-change.

**An end to shame.** Just as a woman's natural body functions had been called abnormal—menstruation was "the curse"; menopause, a "partial death"—so, too, her cancers were a cause for special anguish. For women, says cancer historian James T. Patterson, cancer was "not only medically lethal but also emotionally devastating. Ashamed, embarrassed, in their minds de-sexed, women with [cancer of the breast] often clung desperately to their awful secret [heightening] a virtual conspiracy of silence that surrounded the disease."

Like every conspiracy, this one lived in darkness, nurtured by a lack of effective detection and treatment. Before the introduction of mammography and CAT scans, few breast tumors were found before they had metastasized. Even when a cancer was discovered early, the only accepted treatment—disfiguring radical mastectomy—was no guarantee of cure.

But in the early seventies, that began to change. In May 1971, at the same national breast cancer conference in Los Angeles where Edward Lewison presented his list of women who might be at higher risk of breast cancer if they used birth control pills, Philip Strax, M.D., of Mt. Sinai Medical Center in New York, described the opening of two clinics in New York City offering the new, ten-minute "xero-mammography" that could identify tumors too small to be felt by an examining hand.

There was also a new and energetic debate about mastectomy, a procedure that had been around, in one form or another, at least since the time of the ancient Greeks.

Hippocrates thought that the only way to cure a cancer was to cut it out; he advocated amputation of a cancerous breast. Galen, the Greek-born physician who named cancer from the Greek and Latin words for crab, accepted surgery for breast tumors but adamantly opposed any operation that removed the pectoral muscles of the chest wall. His view held sway straight on through the Dark Ages of history. Ironically, as journalist Rose Kushner wrote in *Breast Cancer,* the memoir of her ultimately unsuccessful fight against the disease, it took "the bright age of modern medicine to make excision of these chest muscles a routine practice."

The new surgery to remove the breast, the chest muscles, various lymph nodes, and sometimes some ribs as well was invented in England in 1867, twenty-one years after Boston dentist William Morton introduced the anesthesia that made such long and complicated operations possible. But it was popularized by an American, William Stewart Halsted, M.D., who performed his first radical mastectomy at John Hopkins in 1889. By the 1930s, Halsted's procedure had been discredited in Europe, where the modified radical mastectomy, a procedure that left the chest muscles intact, swiftly became the standard.

In 1971, while Fasal and Paffenbarger were collecting their statistics in San Francisco, George Crile, M.D., of the Cleveland (Ohio) Clinic, went to the Los Angeles conference on breast cancer to talk about his strong belief that a "simple" mastectomy that removed the whole breast but left chest muscles intact could be as effective as a radical mastectomy. Crile's own studies, showing that both operations produced the same 70 percent five-year survival rate, were supported three years later by a preliminary report from a nationwide study released in October 1974, less than one month after Betty Ford's radical mastectomy. The results showed that, as Crile had suggested, the simple mastectomy was as effective as the radical in preventing recurrence of the original disease. Today, the Halsted radical has been virtually abandoned in the United States.

These new diagnostic and surgical techniques helped to blow away the veil of secrecy surrounding breast cancer. A third important development was the growing use of new anticancer drugs to fight both an original tumor *and* its potential metastases. By 1974, doctors had come to think of breast cancer as a systemic rather than a localized disease. The surgeons were still removing breasts, but the oncologists now offered post-surgical chemotherapy with the anticancer drug L-phenylalanine mustard (better known by its acronym, L-PAM). There was news of a test to detect chemical "markers" in the blood that could warn of a recurrence of a cancer. And at year's end, in December, the National Cancer Institute reported that clinical trials in progress since 1970 showed promising results with the potent new anticancer drug doxorubicin (Adriamycin), which today is one of the drugs in the basic armament against breast cancer.

Mammography, simple mastectomy, lumpectomy, chemotherapy—the studies, reports, and conferences energized the cancer specialists, while a lengthening list of celebrity victims willing, even eager, to talk about their disease, energized the public.

Actress-turned-diplomat Shirley Temple Black, Senate wives Marvella Bayh and Elizabeth Fulbright, reporter Rose Kushner, First Lady Betty Ford, Margaretta "Happy" Rockefeller, wife of vice president–designate Nelson Rockefeller, television reporter Betty Rollin—this new generation of women with breast cancer was neither ashamed nor embarrassed. They talked about their mastectomies and their feelings. They urged other women to seek mammography. And sometimes they voiced the suspicion that was creeping steadily into the national consciousness, the idea that taking estrogen was somehow related to an increased risk of breast cancer.

When her cancer was diagnosed in October 1971, Marvella Bayh "gathered up reasons" to explain what had happened. "For years I had used estrogen to regulate my cycles," she wrote. "Had that caused my cancer?"

In June 1974, when journalist Rose Kushner's tumor was discovered, she, too, wondered whether estrogens were to blame. "I had never taken birth control pills," she wrote, "but now that I was thinking of The Pill as a female hormone, an estrogen, rather than as a contraceptive, I realized how many times I had been given prescriptions for one estrogen or another: to regulate menstrual periods, to prevent miscarriage, or to 'dry up' after weaning my children from the breast. And who knew how much diethylstilbestrol (DES)—the hormone used to fatten livestock—I have eaten in chopped liver and chicken soup?*

They were not the only ones asking questions about female hormones. If Mrs. Ford and Mrs. Rockefeller never speculated openly, a public information officer at the FDA did it for them. When their cancers were diagnosed, he said, "The first thing that popped into somebody's mind here at FDA was, 'I wonder if they were talking OCs' [oral contraceptives]."

By then, California epidemiologists Ralph Paffenbarger and Elfriede Fasal might well have been wondering the same thing.

---

**Two puzzling conclusions.** In October 1975, Paffenbarger and Fasal published the results of their San Francisco study in the *Journal of the National Cancer Institute.* The article was distinguished by two things the authors called "puzzling."

First, women who had used The Pill for two to four years appeared to have a "significantly increased" risk of breast cancer: 1.9 times the risk of women who had never used oral contraceptives. But the higher risk did not show up among

---

* In August, 1972, the FDA banned the use of DES in cattle and sheep feed (it had been banned in poultry feed since 1959). The ban was overturned by the District of Columbia Federal Court in January 1973, and reinstituted by congressional legislation on September 10, 1975.

women who had used The Pill for longer than four years. Second, women who were healthy when they started taking birth control pills seemed to have a lower risk of developing benign breast disease when they were using oral contraceptives, while women who had undergone a biopsy for benign breast disease before they started taking birth control pills and then used oral contraceptives for six years or longer were six to eleven times more likely than other women to develop breast cancer. The longer the use, the higher the risk.

One possible explanation for these contradictions was that the higher risk among short-term users of The Pill had occurred by chance. Another was that estrogen acted as a tumor promoter, speeding up the growth of existing but undiagnosed lesions that were then detected within two to four years after a woman started using The Pill. If this were true, it would go a long way toward explaining why oral contraceptives seemed to be risky for women with prior breast disease. And it would explain another interesting finding, a higher risk among *current users*—women who were still taking The Pill when their cancer was diagnosed. (This slipped by virtually unnoticed and would show up again in 1989, when a nationwide study of more than 120,000 married, female nurses came up with a similar conclusion.) In any event, Fasal and Paffenbarger said that it would be "ill-advised" to prescribe hormones for women previously diagnosed with benign breast disease.

The reaction to this study was summed up in a comment from NCI epidemiologist Robert Hoover, who said the identification of groups of women at particular risk from The Pill was clearly disturbing to anyone whose familiarity with the epidemiology of breast cancer had already led him to suspect that benign breast disease combined with long-term use of estrogen increased a woman's risk of breast tumors. The appearance of an apparent adverse effect of The Pill among these women, he said, might be "an important warning," because, he adds today, "it was the first study to detail a possible link between The Pill and breast cancer."

In the spring of 1977, having retraced their steps through their 1975 data, Paffenbarger and Fasal published a series of "hypotheses and antitheses" regarding oral contraceptives.

On the one hand, they wrote, when a healthy woman took birth control pills, she was less likely to develop benign breast disease, perhaps because The Pill suppressed her body's natural production of estrogens, including estrone and estriol, which were known carcinogens. On the other hand, oral contraceptives seemed to increase the risk of breast cancer for a woman with *existing* benign breast disease. Finally, oral contraceptives prevented pregnancy, and by now, it was commonly accepted that a woman who put off becoming pregnant until after her thirtieth birthday was at higher risk of breast cancer.

Because these theoretical good and bad qualities of The Pill were not "mutually exclusive," Paffenbarger and Fasal decided that it might be time to ask whether it was "wise for young women to use oral contraceptives to defer their first childbirth."

Between 1977 and 1980 there were four more studies published dealing with the possibility that taking birth control pills might raise a woman's risk of breast cancer. Three showed no connection. One, co-authored by Paffenbarger in 1979, showed a higher risk for women who used birth control pills for longer than one year.

Then, in 1981, biostatistician Malcolm Pike, Ph.D., and a team of researchers from the Department of Family and Preventive Medicine at the University of Southern California School of Medicine in Los Angeles tossed a wild card into the debate about The Pill and breast cancer: age.

## *Younger Women, Higher Risk*

Then, as now, breast cancer was primarily a disease of older women; the risk at age fifty is 200 times the risk at age twenty.

Thus, any evidence that an estrogen product such as birth control pills might be linked to an increase in the risk of breast cancer among younger women would be a discovery of major importance. It would not matter if the number of "extra" cases were small. What would count was that there were *any* extra cases at all.

By 1981 it was clear that the age at which a woman went through her first full-term pregnancy was a critical risk factor for breast cancer. The longer a woman put off having children, the higher her risk. Malcolm Pike took this observation one step further, interpreting it to mean that the adolescent and early adult years were also a critical time for establishing breast cancer risk. If he was right, a woman who

*Table 2.* **Incidence of Breast Cancer Among American Women**

| Age | Number of Cases for Each 100,000 Women |
|:---:|:---:|
| 15–19 | 0.1 |
| 20–24 | 1.0 |
| . . . | . . . |
| 40–44 | 120 |
| . . . | . . . |
| 50–54 | 200 |

Source: Susan Harlap, Kathryn Kost, Jacqueline Dorroch Forrest, *Preventing Pregnancy: Protecting Health.* New York: Alan Guttmacher Institute, 1991.

took birth control pills while she was very young might seriously increase her chances of developing "early onset breast cancer," the term cancer experts often use to describe malignant breast tumors occurring before age forty–forty-five.

To test his theory, Pike focused on 163 breast cancer patients under thirty-five years of age when first diagnosed through the USC Cancer Surveillance Program, the cancer registry for Los Angeles County. In their interviews and medical records he found a strong suggestion that *any* use of oral contraceptives by very young women before a first full-term pregnancy could double the risk of early-onset breast cancer. Using The Pill for more than eight years before a first full-term pregnancy appeared to triple the risk. Thus Pike concluded he had been right: The early reproductive years were, indeed, a "critical period."

Over the next two years the study expanded, eventually ending up with 314 women younger than thirty-seven at the time their cancers were diagnosed (plus 314 healthy women who served as controls). The analysis of the data on this larger group, published in *Lancet* in October 1983, echoed the results of the first study: Long-term use before age twenty-five carried a substantial risk of breast cancer at an early age. After one year on The Pill, a young woman's risk of early onset breast cancer was 30 percent higher than normal. After eight years, it nearly quadrupled.

So now there were four studies—two from Paffenbarger, two from Pike—to suggest that using birth control pills at a young age for relatively long periods of time before a first full-term pregnancy significantly increased the risk of breast cancer in women younger than forty.

And everyone knew that from the moment it was introduced, The Pill was extremely popular with young women. Perhaps this was one reason why, as favorable opinion of The Pill among American women rose from 47 percent in 1970 to more than 60 percent in 1980, the number of newly diagnosed cases of breast cancer also went up.

In 1970 there had been 74 newly diagnosed cases a year for every 100,000 women in the United States. By 1980 there were 90.

# chapter 13

# The Official Truth 1980–1987

## Explaining Away the Epidemic

As we have seen, there are two ways to tell how common an illness is in any given population. The first is to measure incidence (the number of new cases each year). The second is to tabulate mortality (the number of deaths).

*Table 3*. **Breast Cancer Trends in America 1940–1980**

|  | DEATHS PER 100,000 WOMEN (APPROX.) | INCIDENCE PER 100,000 WOMEN (APPROX.) | RISK |
| --- | --- | --- | --- |
| 1940 | 28 | 59 | 1-in-20 |
| 1950 | 26 | 65 | 1-in-15 |
| 1960 | 26 | 72 | 1-in-14 |
| 1970 | 27 | 74 | 1-in-13 |
| 1980 | 26 | 90 | 1-in-11 |

Source: American Cancer Society

In the United States, the annual number of deaths from breast cancer remained stable from 1940, when post-menopausal estrogens were first introduced into the general population, through the 1960s, when birth control pills appeared, and straight on to 1980. But the incidence and risk of breast cancer continued to climb.

Faced with this unexplained, steady increase in cases of breast cancer and challenged by the Pike and Paffenbarger studies from California, the contraceptive establishment that had defended The Pill during the blood-clot-and-lawsuit scare before and after the Nelson hearings once again circled its wagons.

The most powerful branch of the establishment was the federal government. In 1960, the Food and Drug Administration had approved The Pill based on the scanty data from Puerto Rico (and had *never* required any trials of ERT). Now, seeking to repair the damage and gain control of the debate about The Pill and cancer, two other federal agencies—the U.S. Centers for Disease Control (CDC) in Atlanta and the National Institute of Child Health and Development (NICHD) in Washington—moved to establish an authoritative central source of information on the subject.

In December 1980, just before the chief epidemiologist in the CDC's Family Planning Evaluation Division announced that the benefits of birth control pills outweighed their risks and pronounced The Pill the "safest and most advantageous form of birth control for those under 30," the CDC joined forces with NICHD's Center for Population Research to create the Cancer and Steroid Hormones Study (CASH), a case/control project to examine the possibility of a link between the use of birth control pills and the rising incidence of reproductive cancers.

Between December 1980 and December 1982, the CASH investigators used information from the National Cancer Institute's SEER centers in metropolitan Atlanta, Detroit,

San Francisco–Oakland, and Seattle, the entire states of Connecticut, Iowa, and New Mexico, plus four urban counties in Utah to identify 5,884 cases, women age twenty to fifty-four at the time their cancers were first diagnosed. Eighty percent of these women (4,730) agreed to be interviewed. During the same two-year period, 5,698 healthy women living in the same geographic areas were identified through random-dialed telephone calls, and 83.4 percent of these cancer-free women (4,754) agreed to serve as controls.

The CASH scientists interviewed both the cases and controls, read through their records, and amassed a wealth of data that have subsequently served as a major resource for numerous teams of CDC and NICHD epidemiologists who have continued to dig away at the material, coming at the relationship between birth control pills and breast cancer first from one angle, then from another. Not every analysis they produced included the data from every woman in the study, but until 1987 every report they published appeared to refute Malcolm Pike's proposition that young women who used birth control pills were at higher risk of breast cancer. In fact, they denied the possibility of any link at all between The Pill and cancer.


## Four Analyses, One Conclusion

In December 1982 the first analysis of the CASH interviews showed that, overall, women who used birth control pills for eleven years or more were 10 percent less likely than nonusers to develop breast cancer. Neither a family history of breast cancer nor a personal history of benign breast disease seemed to have any effect on an individual woman's risk.

At first it had seemed that using The Pill before a first full-term pregnancy might produce a 90 percent increase in risk. But when the analysts took into consideration how old the women using birth control pills were when they became pregnant for the first time, and then compared them to nonusers who became pregnant at the same age, the risk for pill-users was only 30 percent above the norm, and there was a different explanation: Delayed pregnancy rather than pill use. So they concluded that using The Pill was no more hazardous than sexual abstinence or marrying late, either of which might also delay a first pregnancy.

In November 1985 a second CASH analysis lent "statistical stability" to the conclusion that using birth control pills did not raise the risk of early breast cancer. In fact, when the author, NICHD's Bruce V. Stadel, M.D., M.P.H., compared pill use with other risk factors, he found strong evidence "overall" that pill use in the United States had no effect on breast cancer risk, and he was "reasonably confident" that there was no cause for continued concern.

Nine months later, in August 1986, deep into the summer of a year in which the American Cancer Society predicted that more than 123,000 women in the United States would be diagnosed with breast cancer and 39,900 would die of the disease, a third CASH analysis appeared. This time, a group of CDC epidemiologists including Phyllis Wingo, M.S., and the principal CASH investigator, Howard W. Ory, M.D., had searched through the records to see whether the different forms and doses of estrogens in various brands of oral contraceptives had different effects on the risk of breast cancer.* The answer was, No. No overall increase in breast cancer among pill users versus nonusers, no greater incidence of breast cancer that could be tied to one form or dose of estrogen.

---

* The estrogens compared in this study were ethinyl estradiol (30 mcg, 35 mcg, 50 mcg) and mestranol (50 mcg, 60 mcg, 75 mcg, 80 mcg, 100 mcg).

In December 1987, Stadel published another report, this time co-authored by James J. Schlesselman, Ph.D., of the Department of Preventive Medicine and Biometrics at the Uniformed Services University in Bethesda, Maryland. The two, looking for the effects of long-term pill use on young women, found no support for Malcolm Pike's theory of high risk at an early age. But the information on women in the subgroups most at risk (those who had used The Pill for a long time before becoming pregnant and those old enough to be in a naturally high-risk group) were very limited. So while they said their results were "generally reassuring," Stadel and Schlesselman could not call them conclusive.

For several years, the sheer size of the CASH project and the quality of the people doing the analyses seemed to preclude serious criticism, even though there were two areas of special concern, elements in the study that might have affected its outcome: using "random dial" telephone calls to select the controls, and measuring the riskiness of birth control pills for its population as a whole rather than for specific subgroups.

The CASH studies, which carried the imprimatur of two agencies of the U.S. government, were repeatedly cited as incontestable proof of estrogen's safety, and for a little more than four years after the first CASH report was published in 1982, the mainstream of epidemiological data continued to exonerate birth control pills as a cause of breast cancer.

Then, in September 1986, the tide began to turn with a steady rushing flow of studies linking birth control pills to a sharply increased risk of cancer among specific groups of women: the very young, those currently using The Pill, and those who had used oral contraceptives for long periods of time.

# chapter 14

# Real Risk, Real Victims 1986–1991

## *Long-Term Users Are at Risk*

In science, a single startling experimental result or a study pointing to an exciting new development can make the headlines, but to make the grade with peer review, the result or study has to be replicable. If it doesn't show up when other scientists run the same experiment, or if other epidemiologists thumb through the same numbers without coming to the same conclusion, then it simply won't be taken seriously. Nor should it.

Straight through the early 1980s, epidemiologists looking for a link between birth control pills and breast cancer were tantalized by Malcolm Pike's idea that birth control pills were risky for young women. But the CASH data did not support Pike's theory. In fact, two CASH analyses—one by Stadel in 1985, and one from Stadel and Schlesselman in 1987—specifically repudiated it. So you can imagine the excitement when, in the three-year period from 1986 to 1989, five major studies appeared from five different countries on three separate continents, each one confirming Pike's observation of a higher risk of breast cancer among young women who took birth control pills for long periods of time.

**Five supporting studies.**   The first endorsement came from Scandinavia, where as many as 77 percent of all fertile Swedish women and 44 percent of all fertile Danish women had used The Pill at one time or another. The researchers interviewed 422 breast cancer patients younger than forty-five and 722 healthy women of the same age. They found a significantly increased risk of breast cancer among women who used The Pill for a long time while young. The odds began to rise after seven years, but the true flash point occurred at twelve years, when the risk of breast cancer doubled.

Soon there was another study with a similar conclusion. In New Zealand, a national survey showed that early breast cancer was most likely to occur among young women who used The Pill for ten years or more.

None of this new evidence swayed The Pill's defenders, who held staunchly to their position. In December 1987, for example, Louise Tyrer, M.D., vice president for medical affairs of the Planned Parenthood Federation of America, sent a strong memo to executive and medical directors of the Planned Parenthood affiliates justifying the decision by the organization's National Medical Committee not to recommend any changes in the use of oral contraceptives. The new surveys, she said, were inconclusive. Better to rely on the Cancer and Steroid Hormones Study, the "largest and most comprehensive published investigation in the world." It, said Tyrer, was "reassuring, particularly for women in the U.S.A."

But by the time the Tyrer memo was distributed, even the CASH epidemiologists were beginning to pull back from the absolute certainty that had characterized their early analyses. In the fall 1987 issue of Planned Parenthood's own *Medical Digest*, Phyllis Wingo acknowledged the continuing debate among epidemiologists regarding the risks of pill use and

called the then-current state of knowledge "less than satisfy-
ing." "Large numbers of women who were born in the 1940s
and used OCs [oral contraceptives] in the 1960s will begin to
reach the ages at high risk for breast cancer by the year
2000," she said. "Therefore, if OC use at young ages
promotes breast cancer, and if at least 20 years is required
between exposure to OCs at young ages and the diagnosis of
breast cancer, then these women might be expected to be
diagnosed with breast cancer sometime during the next 20
years. Under these assumptions, researchers may not yet be
able to detect such a relationship."

But within four months, they had.

In March 1988, CASH investigators Stadel and Schlesselman, who only a year earlier had been "reasonably confident" that there was no link between oral contraceptives and
breast cancer, published a new analysis of the CASH data.
The new findings showed an increased risk of breast cancer
among childless women who had their first menstrual period
before age thirteen, started taking birth control pills before
age twenty, and stayed on The Pill for more than eight years.
For these women, the risk of early-onset breast cancer was a
stunning 5.6 times higher than the norm.

Next, in May 1989, the U.K. National Case-Control Study
Group—scientists from Oxford University, the Institute of
Cancer Research, and the Imperial Cancer Research Fund,
where Malcolm Pike was temporarily in residence—threw its
considerable weight behind the long-term use/higher-risk
theory.

The study included 755 of the 1,049 breast cancer patients
in eleven geographic areas in Great Britain who were
younger than thirty-six when their tumors were diagnosed
between December 1, 1982, and December 31, 1985, plus an
equal number of controls. When the British interviewed
these women, they found a 43 percent increase in the risk of
breast cancer among those who had used birth control pills

for at least four years. After eight years, the risk was 74 percent higher than normal, and the documentation was so thorough that the Britons were willing to step forward as the first epidemiologists to name the specific number of cases caused by The Pill. If their data were correct, 209 breast tumors, *1 out of every 5 breast cancers recorded in the British National Study,* could be attributed to the use of oral contraceptives.

After that, it was almost an anticlimax when a 1989 Swedish study from University Hospital in Lund showed that using The Pill for three to five years before age twenty-five doubled the risk of early-onset breast cancer. Among women who took The Pill for more than five years before age twenty-five, the risk was 5.3 times the expected rate.

---

**What these numbers mean.**   Identifying long-term use of birth control pills as a significant risk factor was a crucial turning point in the search for a link between The Pill and breast cancer. It could explain why earlier studies counting everyone together, women who had used The Pill for a month along with women who had used it for ten years, had found no increase in risk. And it offered the promise of an easy, practical way to reduce the risk of breast cancer in young women simply by limiting the length of time they stayed on birth control pills.

So these five confirming studies made a lot of people wonder why CASH, with its steady government funding and wealth of cases, hadn't found the same thing.

One explanation is that CASH was flawed by the way in which it selected its controls, the healthy women to whom the breast cancer patients were compared.

In Paffenbarger and Fasal's study of birth control pills and breast cancer or benign breast disease among patients in San Francisco–area hospitals, both the cases and the controls were hospital patients, clearly identified and easily interviewed. The CASH cases were also clearly identified, breast cancer patients in the SEER centers, but the controls were selected by random-dialed telephone calls.

Today, CASH scientists argue that where telephone ownership is high, telephone-based sampling can yield a nearly random sample of people in the population. They are right—so long as the selection really is random, which means that everyone you call answers the phone and answers your questions. But if some of the women who used birth control pills did not do that, then as one CASH epidemiologist admits, "The reported estimates of risk [would] be incorrect. Since we did not have histories of oral contraceptive use for the women we called, we were unable to directly assess the magnitude of this type of bias."

That is what some critics feared. "We were never told how many screening interviews were done to identify the healthy women invited to participate, so the 5,698 healthy women were not really the random sample they are purported to have been," says Graham Colditz, M.D. of Harvard Medical School.

A second explanation for CASH's failure to identify a higher risk of breast cancer among young women using The Pill might be the fact that for several years CASH analyses concentrated on the overall risk for all the women in the study. The first serious analysis of the effects of The Pill on specific groups of women in the CASH sample did not appear until 1988, when Bruce Stadel and James Schlesselman found a nearly sixfold increase in risk among young women who had used birth control pills for long periods of time.

As for CASH's measuring risk for its population as a whole rather than for specific groups of women, Robert Hoover, who is today chief of the environmental epidemiology branch of the National Cancer institute, reminds us that CASH came along early in the game, when "people were looking at the effect of The Pill overall and finding nothing. It was only when they started to look at young women and then young women who had used The Pill for extended time before becoming pregnant, that they began to see something. But subgroup analyses are hard to pin down. You find something, and then someone finds something else, and even in the positive studies, the ones that show a result, it's not always clear. CASH analyzed to beat the band; they did a good job with what they had."

## Current Users: Still at Risk

In 1975, Paffenbarger and Fasal had found an increased risk of breast cancer among "current users" of The Pill, a category they defined as women who were still using The Pill when their cancer was diagnosed. Now, fourteen years later, the Nurses Health Study in Boston was about to release a report showing a similarly increased risk of breast cancer among current users of The Pill.

The Nurses Health Study is the largest, longest-running project designed specifically to examine women's health issues. Created in 1976 by a team of researchers from Harvard Medical School, Harvard School of Public Health, and Brigham and Women's Hospital (Boston), it is named for its participants, 121,700 married female registered nurses in eleven states who completed and mailed in detailed questionnaires about known and suspected risk factors for cancer and heart disease. Once they joined the study, the women tended to stay with it. Every two years, a new questionnaire was mailed out; by 1986, 97 percent of the nurses who were past or current pill users and 93 percent of those who had never used oral contraceptives had continued to update their medical histories and mail in their forms.

When the study started, most (118,273) of the thirty- to fifty-five-year-old women in the sample had no history of cancer other than nonmelanoma skin cancer. By 1985, there were 1,799 newly diagnosed cases of breast cancer among the nurses. Like CASH, the 1985 Nurses Health Study Report and a second one in 1989 showed no apparent increase in risk overall among long-term users of The Pill, even among women who had taken oral contraceptives for as long as four years. Nor was the risk higher than normal for women in their mid-forties and fifties who had used oral contraceptives at some time in the past or while they were very young or before a first full-term pregnancy.

But nestled in among the soothing observations in the 1989 report was a red flag for "current users" (now defined as women who used birth control pills until at least two years before their cancer was diagnosed). In this group, the risk of malignant breast tumors was 60 percent higher than expected; in an even more specific subgroup, current users age forty to forty-four, it was 166 percent higher.

For people who believe that taking estrogens raises the risk of reproductive cancers, the big question had always been whether the hormones initiated new tumors or promoted the growth of existing ones. The discovery of a higher risk of breast cancer among current pill users in the Nurses Health Study seemed to suggest the latter. So did the discovery that the nurses who developed breast cancer while using The Pill were more likely to have tumors that had metastasized by the time they were found, and more likely as well to have tumors that grew in response to estrogen.

---

**Positive proof?**  As we have already seen, in the years immediately after sex hormones were isolated and identified, there were several attempts to use them to treat breast cancer. At first, doctors tried the male hormone testosterone, a logical choice given the fact that removing a premenopausal breast cancer patient's ovaries, the major source of female hormones, often slowed the progress of her disease.

Early on, there were some partial successes with testosterone. It did not cure advanced breast cancer, but it did relieve the pain of metastases to the bones. There was no such good news about female hormones. Despite repeated attempts, no one was able to show that administering either ovarian extracts or estrogens affected the course of breast cancer. But then, in 1944, a team of English researchers reported having shrunk post-menopausal breast tumors with estrogens, and in 1946, a *New York Times* story from the annual meeting of the American College of Surgeons in Cleveland said that estrogen had "influenced a reduction in the mass of a breast cancer [that approached] total elimination of the disease."

Logic says that this cannot have been true. On the contrary, if removing a woman's ovaries could make a cancer shrink, then adding estrogen should make it grow. And in fact, says Gerald Murphy, M.D., chief medical officer of the American Cancer Society, using estrogens to treat breast cancer produced no benefits.

There was, it turned out, a simple explanation for this.

Modern oncologists know that a certain percentage of breast cancers—one study of 1,100 women put the number at 30 percent—contain estrogen receptors, cell chains that hook up with estrogen molecules. Tumors that contain these cell chains are called estrogen receptor-positive (ER+).

ER+ tumors normally grow when exposed to estrogen and shrink when their source of estrogen disappears. Thus, says Dr. Murphy, the development in 1975 of the estrogen receptor assay, a test that pinpoints the presence of estrogen receptors in tumor tissue and allowed doctors to identify estrogen-dependent tumors, "sounded the death knell for the use of estrogens to treat breast cancers."

Now the discovery of an increase in estrogen-responsive tumors among pill-users in the Nurses Health Study and the observation of an increased risk of breast cancer among "current users" appeared to validate the idea that estrogen promoted the growth of existing lesions.

Seven months later, in April 1990, Robert Hoover, M.D., of the National Cancer Institute and Andrew G. Glass of the Center for Health Research at Kaiser-Permanente in Portland, Oregon, added fuel to this epidemiological fire with a study showing that, based on information from the Kaiser-Permanente tumor registry for the United States, the incidence of ER+ breast tumors nationwide had gone up 131 percent between 1974 and 1985, nearly five times faster than the incidence of tumors without estrogen receptors. The highest increase was among women over sixty—that is, the women old enough to have used both birth control pills and ERT.

But was The Pill (or ERT) to blame?

Hoover isn't sure. "The hypothesis that the increase in ER+ tumors is due to hormonal influences is an attractive one, but we have been unable to prove it," he says. "Some people think that the increase is a factor of early detection. Their theory is that all breast cancers start out containing estrogen receptors and lose [the receptors] when they start to go haywire—in other words, the earlier you find these tumors, the more ER+ ones there will be."

As this is written, the reason for the increase in the number of ER+ tumors remains a mystery. But the higher incidence of breast cancer among women currently using The Pill was reconfirmed in June 1991 when the World Health Organization (WHO) published the results of its hospital-based, case/control project, the Collaborative Study of Steroid Contraceptives.

The WHO study covered three developed countries (Australia, the German Democratic Republic, and Israel), and seven developing ones (Chile, China, Kenya, Mexico, Nigeria, the Philippines, and Thailand). Among women currently using birth control pills, the incidence of breast cancer was, on average, 60 percent higher than it was for nonusers. The increase in risk was slightly lower (40 percent) for women who had been using The Pill only for a year or two, but for women whose current use exceeded nine years, the risk was 100 percent higher than it would have been without The Pill.*

## Even Those Who Disagree Agree

By the end of 1990 the statistical evidence of a link between birth control pills and breast cancer in the very young or those who used The Pill long-term was so strong that a CDC "meta-analysis" in the December issue of *Cancer,* comparing the results of twenty-nine previous studies on birth control pills, showed a 50 percent increase overall in the risk of early-onset breast cancer among young women using birth control pills for ten years or more.

Four months later, in April 1991, the Alan Guttmacher Institute published a report called *Preventing Pregnancy, Protecting Health: A New Look at Birth Control Choices in the United States.*

The Guttmacher Institute is what you might call a charter member of the contraceptive establishment. It was created in

---

* Unlike the nurses study, the WHO project also showed an elevated risk for past users, but the higher risk didn't seem to last forever. Women who had stopped using oral contraceptives nine or more years before the survey was done were actually 10 percent less likely than nonusers to develop breast cancer.

1968 as the research, policy analysis, and education arm of the Planned Parenthood Federation of America. Then, in 1977, it was incorporated as a separate, independent agency serving as a "special affiliate" of PPFA. Today, Guttmacher publishes *Family Planning Perspectives,* a well-respected journal that addresses social research issues in contraception, and *Washington Memo,* which covers public policy and government issues.

Like the rest of its establishment brethren, Guttmacher has always defended The Pill. That's what it intended to do with *Preventing Pregnancy,* whose message was neatly captured in a newspaper headline reading, "Safe Sex, Safe Contraception."

But the headline was misleading on both counts.

By 1991 the popular definition of "safe sex" was intimate behavior that protected against AIDS and other sexually transmitted diseases (STDs). As the Guttmacher study correctly notes, birth control pills do seem to protect against one STD— pelvic inflammatory disease. But The Pill does not inhibit the transmission of other STDs such as chlamydia, gonorrhea, syphilis, and AIDS. In fact, there is evidence to suggest that it may alter the climate of the female reproductive tract so as to make a woman more susceptible to infection.

Second, and more important, while the Guttmacher data do indicate a lower incidence of all "reproductive cancers" among pill users, this is true only if you think of three distinct diseases—cancer of the ovary, endometrial cancer, and breast cancer—as a single illness called "reproductive cancer." As soon as you separate out the figures on breast cancer, the picture changes: Ovarian and endometrial cancer *are* still less common among women using the The Pill, but breast cancer is *more* common.

This is a compelling point, says Harvard's Graham Colditz, because the only way to get an accurate view of The Pill's relationship to cancer is to describe the difference between the total cancer incidence—that is, all female reproductive cancers—among pill users. In such an analysis, the risks and benefits are weighed against each other as the incidence of site-specific cancers such as breast cancer, ovarian cancer, or cancer of the uterus are all considered.

Read in this light, *Preventing Pregnancy* does not exonerate The Pill. On the contrary, it strongly indicates that long-term use of oral contraceptives may increase the risk of breast cancer among young women. Furthermore, based on the figures cited in the report, it is entirely possible to put a real number to the risk, to estimate exactly how many "extra" cases of breast cancer will occur due to The Pill.

Statistics cited in *Preventing Pregnancy* compare the incidence of breast cancer among American women who have used The Pill for ten years or more versus those who never used The Pill. Among users and nonusers age fifteen to twenty-four, the numbers are identical: No breast cancers at all among women age fifteen to nineteen; one case for each 100,000 women age twenty to twenty-four. But at age twenty-five to twenty-nine, when breast cancer is ordinarily uncommon, there are 50 percent more cases of breast cancer among long-term pill users. At age thirty to thirty-four, there are 43 percent more. At age thirty-five to forty, when the percentage of women using oral contraceptives begins to decline, the incidence of breast cancer is still 11 percent higher among pill users. At age forty to forty-four, the incidence of breast cancer remains 10 percent higher among women who have used The Pill. Not until after age forty-five, when many women are approaching menopause, pill use is extremely rare, and *the natural incidence of breast cancer begins to climb steeply,* do the numbers turn around to show more cases of breast cancer among women who have never used oral contraceptives. Among women over forty-five, breast cancer is 10 percent *less common* among those who have used birth control pills.

**Hard numbers.**    Until 1989 the numbers cited in studies of The Pill and breast cancer described the increase in risk women might run into when they used oral contraceptives. The 1989 U.K. National Case-Control Study was the first to quantify the increase in risk by actually estimating the number of cases that might occur because of pill use.

The numbers in the Guttmacher study show how many "extra" cases of breast cancer would occur among every 100,000 American women using The Pill. But how many "extra" cases would that be overall, throughout the entire country, for one year?

To find out, you need one more piece of information: How many women in each age group are actually using The Pill. For that you can go to another pillar of the contraceptive establishment, Ortho Pharmaceuticals.

Ortho is the leading marketer of birth control pills in the United States. Since 1968 the company has published an annual study on pill use in this country. According to the twenty-third edition, released four months after the Guttmacher study was published, 15 percent of all American women age fifteen to seventeen used birth control pills in 1990. Among women age eighteen to twenty-four, the number is 49 percent; at age twenty-five to twenty-nine, 38 percent; at age thirty to thirty-four, 23 percent; at age thirty-five to thirty-nine, 10 percent; at age forty to forty-four, 4 percent. (There was no information on pill use among women over forty-five.)

As noted, young women are by nature much less likely than older women to develop breast cancer. For every two hundred breast cancer patients age fifty to fifty-four, there is only one breast cancer patient age twenty to thirty. Since 1981, Malcolm Pike had argued that using birth control pills would upset this balance and increase the risk to young

*Table 4.* **The Pill and Breast Cancer**

| AGE | 15–17 | 18–24 | 25–29 | 30–34 | 35–39 | 40–44 | 45–49 |
|---|---|---|---|---|---|---|---|
| Cases per 100,000 American women who used The Pill for 10 yrs or more* | 0 | 1 | 9 | 30 | 68 | 123 | 169 |
| Cases per 100,000 women who never used The Pill* | 0 | 1 | 6 | 21 | 61 | 112 | 188 |
| Incidence of cancer, users v. nonusers | — | — | 50% higher | 43% higher | 11% higher | 10% higher | 10% lower |
| Number of pill users this age bracket [in 000s]† | 731 | 6,429 | 4,034 | 2,526 | 1,006 | 356 | (NA) |
| Excess cases of breast cancer among pill users‡ | — | — | 121 | 227 | 70 | 39 | (NA) |

* Susan, Harlap, Jacqueline Darroch Forrest and Kathryn Kost. *Preventing Pregnancy: Protecting Health.* New York: The Alan Guttmacher Institute, 1991.

† Based on population data from U.S. Department of Commerce, Bureau of the Census, 1990; and Ortho Pharmaceutical Corp. estimates of the percentage of women in each age group using The Pill.

‡ Based on data from Census, Ortho, and Guttmacher estimates of incidence per 100,000 women

women. The CDC's meta-analysis of twenty-nine studies supported him. Now the Guttmacher study did, too.

Based on the estimates of the incidence of breast cancer among pill users cited in *Preventing Pregnancy* and the Ortho estimates of the percentage of women using The Pill, it is clear that long-term use of birth control pills appears to raise the risk of breast cancer for women age twenty-five to forty-four.

In fact, the numbers cited in the Guttmacher study show that at least 457 cases of breast cancer every year among women younger than forty-five can be attributed to the use of oral contraceptives.

While the number is small—only 3 of every 1,000 cases of breast cancer among American women in 1990—it is significant beyond measure.

Despite repeated disclaimers and the constant assurance that the benefits of oral contraceptives outweigh their risks, the Guttmacher report demonstrates beyond doubt the existence of a potential link between birth control pills and an increased risk of breast cancer.

Now, even those who most vigorously defended The Pill have offered up proof of its dangers.

# ERT and Breast Cancer

# chapter 15

# No Protection
# 1976-1981

## *Building a Case Against ERT*

In *Feminine Forever,* Robert Wilson made a name for himself by insisting that estrogen therapy would protect older women against reproductive cancers. By the end of 1975, the West Coast studies had put the lie to this as far as endometrial cancer was concerned. Then, five months before Paffenbarger and Fasal published their San Francisco study showing increased risk of breast cancer in young women using birth control pills, there were distinct rumblings about a link between ERT and breast cancer as well.

The first indictment was legal, not medical. In May 1975, a New Jersey man went into federal court in Newark with a $2 million lawsuit charging a drug company, Mead Johnson, with negligence in the death of his wife, who had taken birth control pills for six weeks in 1967 to ease her menopausal symptoms. She died of breast cancer in 1973, and now her husband was seeking damages from Mead Johnson because the company had not published a warning about The Pill and breast cancer.

Then, in testimony before the U.S. Senate Subcommittee on Health on January 21, 1976, NCI epidemiologist Robert Hoover mentioned a soon-to-be-published report that would, for the first time, link ERT to an increased risk of breast cancer.


## *One Private Practice*

Like Malcolm Pike, whose questions and theories had framed the debate about The Pill and breast cancer, Robert Hoover played a leading role in the search for a statistical connection between estrogen replacement therapy and breast cancer. His interest in the subject was spawned at Harvard Medical School in the late 1960s, where he studied epidemiology with Brian MacMahon, who, in 1969—along with another Harvard professor, Philip Cole—had told the First National Conference on Breast Cancer that there was indirect evidence from animal tests to connect estrogen to breast cancer. "I was assisting with a large mail survey on birth control pill use in the Boston area," Hoover says, "and as I worked, I was struck with a general concern that [The Pill] was potent hormonal exposure being given to women [when] it was clear that breast cancer was a hormonal disease."

Over the years, MacMahon and Laman D. Gray, Sr., M.D., of the University of Louisville School of Medicine had run into each other at various seminars and conferences. "Gray would give his clinical impression that estrogens were perfectly safe," MacMahon recalls, "and I wouldn't exactly respond since he had one point of view and I had another, which was not that there was something to worry about, but that there were reasons to be cautious. Finally, I got a letter from Gray saying, why don't you come down and study my practice. I asked Bob Hoover, who was now at the National Cancer Institute, to go."

Hoover welcomed what soon turned out to be a serendipitous opportunity to study estrogen's effects on older women. In Louisville, he struck epidemiological gold.

The Kentucky study ran in the August 19, 1976, issue of the *New England Journal of Medicine*. It was a detailed review of the records of 1,891 menopausal women for whom Gray had prescribed conjugated estrogens as hormone replacement therapy in the period from 1939 to 1972. All the women were white; all took estrogens by mouth for at least six months, some for as long as fifteen years.

Based on the current incidence rates among white women in the southern United States, Hoover had expected to find thirty-nine cases of breast cancer among Gray's patients. Instead, he found forty-nine, and when he calculated the difference, it translated to an average 30 percent increase in risk for women who used estrogens as long as ten to fourteen years; using hormones for fifteen years doubled a woman's risk of breast cancer. There was also trouble for women who took 1.25 mg or 2.5 mg estrogen a day, rather than the "standard" 0.3 mg to 0.625 mg. After ten years, their risk of breast cancer was three times that of women who had never taken hormones. (For unknown reasons, women who used estrogens from time to time, rather than on a daily schedule, were also at higher risk.)*

Long-term use of estrogens also seemed to cancel out the protective effect of ovariectomy and make some forms of benign breast disease a more dangerous risk factor. After ten years on ERT, women whose ovaries had been removed by

---

* One interesting anomaly was the fact that in the short term, ERT appeared to be modestly protective. The statistics had predicted fourteen cases of breast cancer among women who took estrogens for less than five years; Hoover actually found thirteen. But, he says, "that could have happened by chance, so it never seemed very important to me. If physicians are doing a pretty good breast exam before a woman goes on ERT and screening out a number of early cases of breast cancer, you would almost always expect to see fewer cancers than predicted among these women in their first few years on estrogen."

hysterectomy—something that ordinarily reduced the risk of breast cancer—were as likely as women who still had their ovaries to be diagnosed with breast tumors. Women who developed benign breast disease *after* they started taking estrogens were seven times more likely to get breast cancer than were women with benign breast disease who had never used hormones.

It wasn't just the numbers that made these findings so striking. It was also their high statistical credibility.

---

**Probability.**   One way to determine whether a statistical result is accurate is to see if it is replicable, which is to say, whether other epidemiologists will come up with the same conclusion when they examine the data. A second way is to assess probability, the possibility that something may happen in the future based on its occurrence under similar conditions in the past.

Probability is often written as an abbreviation: $P$ or $P$ value. The $P$ value measures on a scale of 0-to-1 how likely it is that a particular result occurred simply by chance. A $P$ value of 5 percent (written: 0.05) means that there is only a 5 percent likelihood that the result would have occurred by chance. When a finding has a $P$ value lower than 0.05, it is a pretty good bet that it represents something new and unusual, something you can describe as "statistically significant."

On the other hand, nothing but death and taxes is absolutely certain, so even a $P$ value of 0.05 carries the 1-in-20 possibility that the result occurred by chance. But a low $P$ value is clearly more reassuring than a high one, and a very low $P$ value—less than 0.01—is better yet. As you might expect, scientists hate to produce studies that show no such special effect. What they all look for is a result with a very low $P$ value. Sometimes they look very hard. "If you do enough subset analyses, if you go through 20 subsets, you can find one [such as] the effect of [breast cancer] chemotherapy on pre-menopausal women with [metastases to] two to five lymph nodes. People do this," one experienced scientist told *Washington Post* science reporter Victor Cohn, author of *News & Numbers,* a layman's guide to statistics.

But Hoover had come by the Kentucky numbers honestly. The projection of a 30 percent increase in risk after ten to fourteen years on ERT had a *P* factor of 0.06, just outside the magic 0.05 circle. The estimate of a 100 percent increase in risk after fifteen years of estrogen therapy had a *P* factor of 0.01, an excellent indication that this was not a chance occurrence.

Clearly, menopausal estrogens did not protect a woman from cancer of the breast. Yet Hoover and his co-authors— Gray, Cole, and MacMahon—would not take the next step and say that ERT might cause breast cancer. They were, at best, willing to call it "a definite possibility."

*Table 5.* **Risk of Breast Cancer (among selected age groups)**

| Age | Risk of Developing Breast Cancer | Risk of Dying from Breast Cancer |
|---|---|---|
| 20–30 | 0.04 | 0.00 |
| 35–45 | 0.88 | 0.14 |
| 50–60 | 1.95 | 0.33 |
| 65–75 | 3.17 | 0.43 |
| 65–85 | 5.48 | 1.01 |
| 65–110 | 6.53 | 1.53 |

Source: SEER 1985 figures from *The Merck Manual,* 16th ed. Rahway, N.J.: Merck Research Laboratories, 1992, p. 1816.

## A Federal Case

As the incidence of breast cancer continued to rise, there were more cases among women in every age group, from the very young to the very old. But the risk was still many times higher for older women than for young women, and it was logical to assume that a majority of the 89,000 new cases of breast cancer and 33,000 deaths predicted for 1975 would occur among the nation's 31 million post-menopausal women older than forty-five—the very ones now being targeted for ERT. So any association between ERT and breast cancer contained the seeds of an epidemiological disaster.

In September, when the National Institute on Aging sponsored a Consensus Development Conference to evaluate the risks and benefits of ERT for older women, the Conference delegates acknowledged the connection between ERT and endometrial cancer, something they could hardly avoid doing given the information from the Los Angeles, San Francisco, and Seattle studies. They admitted that a similar relationship between estrogens and breast cancer was well documented in laboratory animals, but cautiously noted that a careful review of several well-conducted case/control studies had not shown the same thing in human beings. True, there had been a disquieting, steady increase in breast cancers starting around 1960–1962, just after The Pill was introduced. True, the increase was higher among white women, who were most likely to be using the various estrogen products. But the percentage of women dying from breast cancer had not gone up; the only study tying The Pill to an increased risk of breast cancer was Fasal and Paffenbarger's San Francisco survey with its "puzzling" results; and the only one to link an increase in breast cancer to the use of estrogen at menopause was Robert Hoover's report on Laman Gray's Kentucky practice.

So in the end the Conference waffled, issuing a statement

of frowning interest rather than a forthright warning of dangers ahead: Breast cancer was so common, it said, and the prognosis so poor, that any possible association with estrogen use was a "concern."

Then everyone went home to wait for the next study and the next set of numbers.

## The Price of Pain and Suffering

In business (including the business of medicine), nothing concentrates the mind as efficiently as cash. Particularly cash won through legal action.

When women using estrogens complained about debilitating side effects, their malaise had been dismissed as the result of the original high-estrogen birth control pills or, more insulting, female suggestibility. But when a major pharmaceutical company agreed to a $250,000 out-of-court settlement with the parents of a seventeen-year-old girl who died of vaginal cancer caused by her mother's using the synthetic estrogen DES while pregnant, that was serious business.

Eli Lilly's settlement on January 18, 1980, could not be ignored or wished away. Its importance was underscored two months later when the California Supreme Court ruled that a suit brought by two DES daughters could go forward. The women were seeking $11 million in damages and the establishment of clinics where DES victims could be diagnosed and treated free of charge. The court did not decide whether their claim was valid. The ruling said only that any company that had marketed DES could be held liable for the drug's adverse effects. The decision opened the way for legal action against Abbott Laboratories, Eli Lilly, Rexall Drug, E.R. Squibb, and Upjohn—all of whom had sold the synthetic estrogen. The companies immediately appealed to the U.S. Supreme Court, but the High Court refused to hear the case. The California decision stood, and in February 1981 the New York State Appeals Court dramatically expanded the number of potential suits when it ruled unanimously that a DES daughter could go after *any* company that had sold the synthetic estrogen. The following year the New York court upheld a $492,000 award to a DES daughter who had won her case against Eli Lilly even though she could not prove that Lilly made or sold the pill her mother took.

These decisions were narrow in the sense that they concerned only vaginal cancers resulting from the use of DES by pregnant women. (In 1984, a study published in the *New England Journal of Medicine* showed a 47 percent increased risk of breast cancer among the approximately 4 million women who had used DES to prevent miscarriage.) But putting a legal stamp of approval on the link between one form of estrogen and one kind of cancer in very young women encouraged speculation about other estrogens and other cancers in other groups of women. By 1989 the U.K. National Case-Control Study Group had issued its report that 20 percent of the breast cancers in its survey were due to The Pill, and there would be eight solid studies to support a similar link to ERT.*

## *Eight Years, Eight Studies, One Conclusion*

As far as Ronald K. Ross, M.D., M.S., and Robert Pfeffer, M.D., were concerned, the most logical place to observe the

---

*There were also five studies that found no connection between ERT and an increased risk of breast cancer, but epidemiologists at the CDC considered these to be less reliable than the studies linking the medicine to the cancer.

effects of estrogen on older women was a retirement community, so the two epidemiologists—one from the University
of Southern California School of Medicine, the other from
the University of California, Irvine—picked two communities
in Los Angeles and went to work. Their results, published in
April 1980, looked a lot like Hoover's Kentucky data: a
higher risk for long-term users and for women who took
large amounts of estrogen. Women who used ERT for seven
years or more were 80 percent more likely than nonusers to
develop breast cancer ($P = 0.02$). Those with intact ovaries
who consumed a total of 1,500 mg estrogen—an amount
approximately equivalent to a standard dose of 1.5 mg
conjugated estrogens every day for three years—were 2.5
times more likely to develop breast cancer than were women
who never took estrogens.

A year later, in May 1981, a new report from Robert
Hoover and Louise Brinton, Ph.D., a National Cancer Institute colleague, showed a 20 percent increase in risk for
post-menopausal women with intact ovaries who used ERT
*for any length of time,* a 54 percent average increase for women
who used estrogens *for any length of time* after their ovaries
had been removed through hysterectomy, and a 700 percent
increase for estrogen-users whose ovaries had been removed
and who also had a family history of breast cancer. (Women
who had given birth to three or more children did not
increase their risk by using estrogens, but for women who
had never had a child, using ERT meant a nearly 700 percent
rise in risk.)

In October, Hoover co-authored a study showing that,
overall, women using ERT were 40 percent more likely than
nonusers to develop breast cancer. For women with a family
history of breast cancer, the risk went up 400 percent. But
the highest increase was among women taking estrogen
*during* rather than *after* menopause. Like young women
taking birth control pills, these peri-menopausal (in Greek,

*peri* means "around") women were getting a double dose of hormones—estrogen pills plus the estrogen secreted naturally by their bodies. For these women, using ERT produced a 700 percent increase in the risk of breast cancer.

After that, the studies indicating ERT continued to roll in. A 1984 survey of 119 cases and 119 controls found higher risk among women who use large doses of estrogen or took the hormone after their ovaries had been removed. In 1986, one group of epidemiologists found a higher risk among estrogen users with benign breast disease or a family history of breast cancer; a second blamed long-term use; a third said taking estrogen for *any* length of time was dangerous. In 1987, CASH investigator Phyllis Wingo found a higher risk among women whose ovaries had been removed or who had a family history of breast cancer. In 1988, the eighth study in the series once again blamed long-term use.

As the decade ended, that was one of the major stories about breast cancer. The second was, of course, the lengthening list of studies linking birth control pills to breast cancer in young women. The third was the steadily growing list of victims.

## The Best Medicine

Actress Bette Davis turned seventy-five in April 1983. She had just completed a leading role in the pilot for a new television series called "Hotel," but the prospect of a new career in television ended abruptly one month later when she discovered a lump in her left breast. On June 9, after conferring with her own doctor in Los Angeles, she underwent a radical mastectomy at New York Hospital. The surgery was followed by a stroke and, soon after, by a broken hip. Davis never returned to "Hotel"; her role went to Anne Baxter, the onetime ambitious ingenue in Davis' 1950 classic movie *All About Eve.*

A year later, on June 1, 1984, actress Jill Ireland was handed the same diagnosis and the same prescription. "That I was to have a radical mastectomy instead of a lumpectomy terrified me," she wrote. "God, my cancer had progressed to the point of a complete mastectomy."

As long ago as 1971, at the Second National Conference on Breast Cancer in Los Angeles, the Cleveland Clinic's George Crile had urged surgeons to eschew Halsted's radical mastectomy in favor of a simple mastectomy that removed breast and lymph nodes but left chest muscles intact. When her own tumor was diagnosed three years later, journalist Rose Kushner sought Crile out and, although she eventually agreed to a mastectomy, strongly supported his campaign to make simple mastectomy and, where possible, lumpectomy the treatments of choice for women whose cancers had not metastasized.

These were not yet popular positions in establishment circles. At the Los Angeles conference, Jerome A. Urban, M.D., acting chief of breast service at New York's Memorial Hospital for Cancer and Allied Diseases, called Crile's studies unreliable. A second Memorial surgeon, Arthur Holleb, M.D., agreed. At the American Cancer Society's annual meeting on October 16, 1974, ACS president George P. Rosemond, M.D., reiterated the organization's support for radical mastectomy, but he did admit that the increasing use of mammography and post-operative chemotherapy might eventually reduce the need for the surgery, especially in light of a recent nationwide study in which women with early cancers who were treated by lumpectomy survived as long as women treated by mastectomy. If these results held up and drug therapy proved effective, said NCI's Vincent DeVita, M.D., eventually breast cancer could be treated by simple surgery and post-operative chemotherapy.

It took more than a decade, but in 1985, Crile was finally vindicated when another nationwide study, this one from University of Pittsburgh breast cancer researcher Bernard Fisher, M.D., showed that lumpectomy plus radiation was as effective as mastectomy in preventing the recurrence of early breast tumors. DeVita, now director of the National Cancer Institute, estimated that as many as 60,000 of the 119,000 women expected to be diagnosed with breast cancer in 1985 might be candidates for this new regime.

The list might not have included Jill Ireland, whose cancer had already spread to her lymph nodes by the time it was discovered, but Nancy Reagan probably would have qualified. Yet in October 1987, when her tumor was diagnosed, she opted for mastectomy, and her decision starkly illuminated the terror breast cancer held even for those lucky enough to have found it early. "A lumpectomy seemed too inconclusive," she said, "and I know, given my nature, that I'd be worried to death. There were people, including doctors, who thought I had taken too drastic a step in choosing the mastectomy. The director of the Breast Cancer Advisory Center was quoted in *The New York Times* as saying that my decision had 'set us back ten years.' I resented those statements, and I still do."

Having made her choice, Mrs. Reagan actively encouraged other women to seek mammography. The response was strong enough to produce an up-and-down jog in breast cancer statistics like the one jn 1974–1975 after Betty Ford was diagnosed and millions of women went for their first mammograms. In 1986, the year before Mrs. Reagan's cancer was discovered, the incidence of breast cancer in this country was 106 cases for every 100,000 women. By the end of 1987, there were 112. The following year, the number dropped to 109.6, and by 1989, it was down to 105, just about where it had been before Mrs. Reagan's operation.

But nobody was celebrating, because the "decline" was, in fact, an illusion.

In 1989 the number of cases of breast cancer for every 100,000 American women was 17 percent higher than it had been in 1980: 105 versus 90.

# chapter 16

# Confirming Evidence 1989–1991

## *Proof from Sweden*

By the time the incidence of breast cancer in the United States reached 105 cases for every 100,000 women, the Scandinavian, New Zealand and U.K. National Case-Control studies on oral contraceptives had confirmed that long-term use of birth control pills by young women was a risk factor for breast cancer, and eight studies between 1980 and 1988 had shown a similar risk for long-term use of ERT.

Now something new appeared: A study from a team of Swedish and American epidemiologists detailing the risks not of estrogen replacement therapy but of hormone replacement therapy (HRT), the estrogen/progestin regime designed to reduce the risk of endometrial cancer for women using hormones after menopause.

For six years, Leif Bergkvist, M.D., of University Hospital, Uppsala, and a group of epidemiologists including two Americans (Robert Hoover and Catherine Schairer, M.S., of NCI) had begun collecting and analyzing information about 23,244 women age thirty-five and older who lived in the Uppsala region of Sweden and had filled prescriptions for post-menopausal hormones. By the time the Bergkvist study was ready to be published in the *New England Journal of Medicine* in August 1989, 253 of the women in the cohort had developed breast cancer, and Hoover was able to say with a certain authority that the study added to "the growing body of evidence that long-term use of menopausal replacement hormones increases a woman's risk of breast cancer."

Overall, there was a 10 percent increase in risk among the women in the Swedish cohort using ERT, but that was too small to be considered statistically significant. In Uppsala, as in Kentucky in 1976, the real problem was long-term use. According to Bergkvist, a woman who used estrogen replacement therapy for nine years or more doubled her risk of breast cancer, a prediction he could make with a serious degree of certainty because it carried a $P$ value of 0.002.

The women in the study used three different types of hormone products: an estrogen-progestin combination designed to reduce the risk of endometrial cancer; estradiol, a form of estrogen rarely used in the United States; and conjugated estrogens. The risk of breast cancer rose most quickly among women using combination pills. For them, the risk of breast cancer after only four years on ERT was more than four times what it would have been without the hormones. After six years, women using estradiol were 80 percent more likely to end up with breast cancer. But women who used conjugated estrogens, had no increase in risk, regardless of how long they stayed with ERT.

Did this mean that estrogen plus progestin or estradiol alone were dangerous and conjugated estrogens were safe? Probably not, said Elizabeth Barrett-Connor, M.D., of the University of California, San Diego. In an editorial that ran in the same issue as the Bergkvist study, she pointed out that during the first half of a normal menstrual cycle, the dominant hormone in a woman's body is estrogen, which signals the cells of the endometrium to proliferate in preparation for the implantation of a fertilized egg. After ovulation, the dominant hormone is progesterone. If no fertilized egg implants—and if the woman does not become pregnant—the rising level of progesterone causes cells in the endometrium to stop dividing. Approximately fourteen days after ovulation the excess endometrial tissue sloughs off, producing menstrual bleeding.

But, as Barrett-Conner explained, progesterone does not slow down the division of cells in breast tissue, which continue to multiply rapidly through the second half of the cycle. So adding progesterone to the estrogen used for post-menopausal replacement therapy might theoretically lessen the risk of endometrial cancer, while an estrogen/progestin birth control pill might increase the risk of breast cancer although there was, as yet, no epidemiological support for this theory.

Barrett-Connor, who had published papers on the safety of ERT, noted that some cardiologists already suspected that progestins might negate the heart-healthy effects of estrogen by raising blood levels of low-density lipoproteins (LDLs), the "bad" fat-and-protein particles that carry cholesterol into arteries. So, she said, any link between progestins and breast cancer deserved serious attention.

As for a comparison between estradiol and conjugated estrogens, the latter might have seemed safer because so few of the Swedish women (only 20 percent of the total) were using them and because the doses they took were lower than what was currently prescribed in the United States. But the women in Hoover's Kentucky study had taken *only* conjugated estrogens, and by 1989 *The Merck Index* listed both estradiol and conjugated estrogens as potential carcinogens.

The implications of the Bergkvist study, that *every* form of post-menopausal HRT appeared to be linked to some increase in the risk of breast cancer, reverberated through the epidemiological community.

In her *NEJM* editorial, Elizabeth Barrett-Connor said the

results from Uppsala "could change the way we think about post-menopausal estrogen replacement." I. Craig Henderson, M.D., then a breast cancer researcher and medical oncologist at the Dana-Farber Cancer Institute in Boston and now on staff at the Mt. Zion Medical Center, University of California, San Francisco, cautioned that it was too soon to make a blanket statement on what hormones a woman should take at menopause. But he called the study "a landmark" whose findings about progestins made "biological sense," a statement with which Malcolm Pike agreed. Robert Hoover's colleague Louise Brinton said it was "a hard call." Doctors, she concluded, were becoming "more concerned and a little less optimistic about [estrogen/progestin] therapy."

And when the Nurses Health Study, which had already tied the current use of birth control pills to an increased risk of breast cancer, said the same thing about post-menopausal estrogens in November 1990, the reaction was decidedly edgy.

## Good Risk, Bad Risk

The bad news, said Harvard's Graham Colditz, a leading researcher with the Nurses Health Study, was that "as soon as you start using ERT, your risk goes up." Women using estrogen were 30 to 40 percent more likely than nonusers or past users to develop breast cancer. The older a woman was when she used ERT, the higher her risk. At age fifty-five to fifty-nine, a woman using ERT increased her risk of breast cancer 50 percent; at age sixty to sixty-four, 100 percent.

The good news was that the effect seemed to be reversible

and might, Colditz suggested, fade away within a year after a woman stopped using estrogens. But that was by no means certain, so he urged caution in the use of estrogens.

Not everyone agreed. In fact, two epidemiologists who had been notably edgy about the implications of the Bergkvist study were less convinced by this one. Louise Brinton, who had been disturbed about possible problems with an estrogen/progestin combination, was more sanguine about estrogen alone. Its benefits, she said, still outweighed the risks. I. Craig Henderson said estrogen's apparent ability to induce breast cancer "almost certainly real and almost certainly small. You have to put [the 30 to 40 percent increase in risk from the Nurses Health Study] in perspective in terms of the other risks we live with normally in life. If you have a mother or a sister with breast cancer, your risk will be twice normal; if you also have atypical hyperplasia and fibrocystic breast disease, your risk would be eight to nine times normal."*

These are rational explanations. Estrogen *does* have benefits for some women; it *does* seem to rank lower as a risk factor than a personal or family history of the disease. But they also say a lot about how we weigh competing risks in this country.

In May 1987 the Nurses Health Study had suggested a similar 30 percent increase in the risk of breast cancer among women who consumed more than three drinks of alcohol a week. These results were widely publicized as proof that any consumption of alcohol would raise the risk of breast cancer, even though statisticians from the U.S. Centers for Disease Control found no such effect for moderate drinkers and a 1988 American Cancer Society study that had

---

*According to Graham Colditz, about one woman in a hundred has both conditions.

followed 581,321 American women for more than twelve years showed virtually no difference in risk between female nondrinkers and women who regularly had two drinks a day. Yet as late as 1990, *Newsweek* continued to tell its readers that "even moderate drinking" might raise a woman's risk 50 percent.

The point, says Graham Colditz, is that this country "has had a problem with alcohol at least since Prohibition, so we do see a whole range of [negative] responses whenever alcohol is discussed. In contrast, ERT is regarded as good because it relieves symptoms of menopause."

Or, as Clark W. Heath, Jr., M.D., vice president for epidemiology and statistics at the ACS, put it: "What we're talking about, is a risk in a white hat [estrogen] and a risk in a black hat [alcohol]."

No wonder people were confused.

## Statistical Proof

In the end, the discussion of ERT's role as a risk factor in the breast cancer epidemic always comes down to numbers: the number of women using the hormones, the number of new cancers each year, and the number of studies that show a connection between the two.

In *Feminine Forever,* Robert Wilson wrote enthusiastically about a "select minority" of women using estrogen replacement therapy in the mid-1960s, a number he put (variously) at 6,000, 12,000, and 14,000. Even at its highest, the figure is small in comparison to the 3.5 million American women who were using menopausal hormones by 1989. There is a similarly disproportionate relationship in the number of cases of breast cancer: 63,000 in 1960 versus 175,000 in 1991, the same year a team of epidemiologists from the CDC and Emory University was about to tie the hormone to the cancer through a meta-analysis comparing data from sixteen previous studies, starting with Hoover's in 1976 and ending with Bergkvist's in 1989.

The CDC/Emory meta-analysis produced simple, straightforward conclusions. ERT was a risk factor for breast cancer separate and distinct from all the others such as a family history of breast cancer or benign breast disease or the number of children a woman had delivered. The risk began to climb after five years on ERT. It reached an average high of 30 percent above normal after fifteen years of hormone therapy.

True, some of the information in the meta-analysis came from studies that included pre-menopausal women. True, that might have influenced the results because these women were taking ERT while their own bodies were still secreting relatively normal amounts of estrogen. True, the benefits of estrogen replacement might outweigh the risks for most women. But none of these disclaimers could obscure the fact that the cold, clear statistical increase in risk demonstrated by the meta-analysis translated into the human agony of real cancers for real women.

Therefore, like the British epidemiologists who in 1989 had been willing to attribute 20 percent of the breast cancers discovered by U.K. Case-Control Study to the use of oral contraceptives, the Atlanta scientists were now ready to name the specific number of cases of breast cancer that might be due to ERT.

"On the basis of our estimate," they said, "approximately 4,708 new cases and 1,468 breast cancer deaths would occur each year because of estrogen use."

If they were right, the number of American women who would develop breast cancer in 1991 because they were using

ERT could end up being equal to one-third of all the women (14,000) predicted to be taking ERT in 1967, one year after Robert Wilson published *Feminine Forever* and set off on his national crusade to guarantee eternal femininity through hormone therapy.

# chapter 17

# Defending ERT 1980–1991

## *Aesthetics versus Health*

Despite the epidemiological evidence linking ERT and HRT to an increased risk of breast cancer, there were still solid grounds on which to defend hormone replacement therapy.

The strongest argument in favor of birth control pills was an aesthetic one: Oral contraceptives protected against pregnancy without interfering with sexual spontaneity or requiring a woman to touch her genitals. But estrogen replacement therapy, as the medical establishment was quick to note, produced real, measurable medical benefits for certain groups of women. Not only did it alleviate menopausal symptoms and reverse some age-related cosmetic changes such as dry skin, it also appeared to prevent osteoporosis, the progressive loss of bone density that occurs as we grow older. And it seemed to reduce dramatically a post-menopausal woman's risk of heart attack.

## *Estrogen and Strong Bones*

The first person to suggest that estrogen deficiency might be responsible for the post-menopausal loss of bone density appears to have been endocrinologist Fuller Albright, who posed the theory in the 1940s. To this day, nobody can say with certainty exactly how estrogen helps the body hold on to bone tissue—there is some suspicion that it works by enabling vitamin D to facilitate the body's absorption of calcium—but there are dozens of studies documenting the existence of a direct relationship between high estrogen levels and strong bones.

As early as 1979, gynecologist Lila Nachtigall of New York University School of Medicine and NYU Medical Center, and colleagues had published the results of a study in which eighty-four menopausal patients who were given estrogen and an equal number who took a placebo showed that over a ten-year period the women taking estrogens suffered virtually no bone loss, while the women on placebos continually lost bone and suffered a number of fractures. Over the next decade, the Nachtigall results were replicated by literally dozens of other scientists observing thousands of other women.

A man's bones also become more porous as he gets older, but the situation is worse for women who may lose as much as 40 to 50 percent of bone density compared with an average 20 to 30 percent for men. As a result, women are more susceptible to broken bones, especially hip fractures, which are twice as common among women. Every year in this country, as many as 184,000 people suffer hip fractures. It is a potentially devastating injury. Nearly a quarter of the people over fifty who break a hip do not heal well enough to be able to walk again without assistance; 20 percent may still be in a long-term care facility a year or more later.

Because most articles on health issues for lay people are

published in magazines meant mainly for women, medical conditions that affect women often get wider attention from the press then they do from the medical establishment. As the population of older women expanded, so did the number of fractures related to osteoporosis. By the mid-1980s, osteoporosis was at the top of the magazine medical hit list, a "disease-of-the-week" tucked in-between two older standbys, PMS and TMJ.*

Then, in 1984 an NIH Consensus Development Conference released a statement saying that estrogen was highly effective at preventing bone loss even if a woman didn't start to take it until six years after menopause. This section of the NIH report was widely publicized, but nobody paid much attention to the fact that NIH had targeted its recommendation to a specific audience—white women whose ovaries were removed before age fifty and who had no medical problems, such as a previous history of breast cancer, that would mitigate against the use of estrogens. What captured the attention was NIH's willingness to consider virtually every woman a potential patient. "Women who have a natural menopause also should be considered for cyclic estrogen replacement," the NIH report said, "if they have no contraindications and if they understand the risks and agree to regular medical evaluations. The duration of estrogen therapy need not be limited."

Consumer advocates objected to the indiscriminate use of estrogens. "Women need to know that [only] 25 percent of us will develop osteoporosis, and black women are at even lower risk," said Davi Birnbaum, then head of the Midlife Women's Health Issues section at the National Women's Health Network. "Osteoporosis is a serious disease, but it's

*The initials TMJ—for temporomandibular joint (the hinge at the side of your face that allows your lower jaw to swing open)—have now been replaced with TMD, for temporomandibular joint disease.

being used to seduce women back to estrogen." Some medical experts objected to the unlimited duration of the treatment. "We haven't got sufficient data to show what happens after several decades of estrogen use," Diane Meier, M.D., of Mt. Sinai Medical Center in New York told *The Washington Post.*

Nonetheless, new estrogen products continued to come on line. In September 1986, the FDA granted its approval for Estraderm, CIBA Consumer Pharmaceuticals' new transdermal patch. The patch, which CIBA called "the enlightened approach to menopause," delivered a continual stream of low-dose estrogens through the skin. In 1986, the FDA approved the use of conjugated estrogens for treating osteoporosis, a decision that expanded the potential market for ERT from the relatively small group of women with severe hot flushes to the enormously larger market of post-menopausal women who were now convinced that a broken hip was the inevitable accompaniment of old age.

## Estrogen and Heart Health

Every year, approximately 300,000 American women over fifty die of heart disease. When oral contraceptives went on the market in 1961, it looked as though taking estrogens might make things worse. First there were pill-related blood clots; then, in the mid-1970s, a major British study estimated that women age thirty to thirty-nine who used The Pill were 2.7 times more likely than nonusers of the same age to suffer a heart attack. For women age forty to forty-four, the pill-related increase in risk was 5.7-fold. But by the late 1960s, there was less estrogen in The Pill and, apparently, less danger for women.

Using estrogen replacement therapy never produced the

same kind of vascular problems, and as it became more popular the NIH hastened to absolve ERT of any role in cardiovascular disease, saying that there was no evidence that it would cause either blood clots or stroke.

On the other hand, whether it would *prevent* vascular problems or heart attack in older women was very much an open question. In 1985, Meir J. Stampfer, M.D., of Harvard Medical School issued a report from the Nurses Health Study saying that estrogen therapy lowered the risk of heart disease in post-menopausal women. But a simultaneous report from the Framingham study said precisely the opposite. In the small western Massachusetts city of Framingham, doctors from Boston University School of Medicine were tracking 5,127 healthy men and women to see who got heart disease and why; the conclusion was that taking estrogen increased the risk of heart disease.* These contradictory findings continued to puzzle epidemiologists until 1991 when three major studies appeared to tip the balance in favor of ERT.

The first two were disclosed in May, at the National Heart Association meeting in Orlando, Florida. In a fourteen-year follow-up study from Johns Hopkins Medical Institutions, women who used post-menopausal hormones appeared to be 63 percent less likely to die of a heart attack, while a National Health and Nutrition Survey showed that women who did not use hormones after menopause were twice as likely to die of stroke.

The third favorable report on estrogen, this time from the Nurses Health Study, was published in September. By now, Stampfer had ten years' worth of data on the 48,470 women in the study who were past menopause and had no history of cancer or heart disease when they joined the cohort. Com-

---

*It was the Framingham scientists who discovered that pre-menopausal women have a lower-than-average risk of heart attack and that people with high levels of serum cholesterol seem to be at higher risk.

paring records, Stampfer found that women using estrogen were 44 percent less likely to suffer a heart attack, perhaps because the hormone raised their levels of high-density lipoproteins (HDLs), the "good" fat-and-protein particles that help eliminate cholesterol from the body.

In the United States, a white woman age fifty through ninety-four has about one chance in three of dying from a heart attack. Her chance of dying from breast cancer is about ten times less, 1-in-36.

Stampfer's study did not *prove* that taking estrogen prevented heart attacks. The nurses study had not been randomly designed, with half the women using estrogens and the other half placebos. Instead, the nurses decided on their own whether to take estrogen, and if the ones who opted for ERT were simply in better shape, more aware of health issues, and thus more likely to try a new therapy at the start, they were also likely to be healthier ten years later. It might look as though estrogen kept a woman healthy when in fact it was just the other way around: Healthy women took estrogen.

Nonetheless, when you considered Stampfer's data in tandem with the reports from Johns Hopkins and the National Health and Nutrition Survey, it began to look as though the pendulum that had swung away from estrogen after the continuing reports of endometrial and breast cancers was beginning to swing back the other way.

After reading through the Stampfer analysis, Lee Goldman, M.D., of Brigham and Women's Hospital said in an editorial in the *New England Journal of Medicine* that if he had to make a choice based on its admittedly imperfect data, he would go with ERT, a decision he reached after balancing the risk of heart disease against the risk of breast cancer. Antonio Gotto, M.D., chairman of the department of medicine at Baylor College of Medicine in Houston and a past president of the American Heart Association, agreed. "The medical profession and women themselves have underestimated the importance of cardiovascular disease in females,'' he said. "I have seen in my own practice women who are afraid to take estrogens because of the risk of cancer."

Then someone gave the pendulum another push.

## Heavy Metal

For years, the estrogen/heart disease question had run like this: Young (pre-menopausal) women have a risk of heart attack dramatically lower than the risk for young men. Older (post-menopausal) women have a risk of heart attack similar to the risk for older men. Since the major difference between the two groups of women and between the young women and the young men is the amount of estrogen their bodies are producing, estrogen must be what protects young women against heart attack.

It was a neat theory, but it didn't work when researchers gave estrogen to men in an attempt to even out the difference (see page 11). What's more, it ignored one major difference between men and women and between women who are young and women who have been through menopause: iron.

In September 1992, a team of researchers led by Jukka T. Salonen of the University of Kuopio in Finland, released the results of a study of 1,931 middle-aged Finnish men who had shown no evidence of heart disease when the study began in 1984. For several years, the scientists routinely drew blood samples from the men to test for stored iron and to measure cholesterol levels. At the same time, they estimated dietary iron intake by reviewing the men's records of what they had eaten in the four days before the blood tests.

At the end, it looked as though the amount of cholesterol

in a man's blood was less important than the amount of iron. Regardless of their cholesterol counts, the men with higher iron levels had a higher risk of heart disease.

There were no women in the study, so what does this have to say about the risk of heart attack in older women?

In the absence of any proof, the only choice is speculation. Hemoglobin is an iron-complex in blood that carries oxygen to every cell in your body. Without enough hemoglobin, less oxygen reaches body cells, and the result is the fatigue associated with mild "iron deficiency anemia."

During her reproductive years, a woman loses blood each month when she menstruates; thus a healthy woman of childbearing age almost always can be expected to have a hemoglobin count lower than that of a healthy man of the same age. The "normal" range for adult men is 14 to 18 grams hemoglobin for each decaliter ($\frac{1}{100}$ of a liter) of blood, a statement written as 14–18 g/dl. For women of childbearing age, the normal range is 12 to 16 g/dl.

After menopause, however, when menstruation ceases, so does the monthly flow of blood. As a result, iron levels among post-menopausal women may stabilize. Can it be that this "excess" of iron, rather than a deficiency of estrogen, is what increases an older woman's risk of heart attack?

If that turns out to be true—and right now no one can say whether it will—one of the strongest arguments in favor of hormone replacement therapy will crumble, while the case against the widespread prescription of female hormones for older women will be significantly stronger.

# chapter 18

# The Fatal Connection 1992

## Decades of Cancer

In 1960, when G.D. Searle introduced the first birth control pill, an American woman's lifetime risk of breast cancer was 1-in-14.

Today, when 20 percent of all American women of childbearing age—the highest percentage in history—are using The Pill, the lifetime risk of breast cancer is 1-in-8.

In 1966, when Robert Wilson wrote *Feminine Forever,* the incidence of breast cancer in the United States was about 73 cases for every 100,000 women. Today, when nearly 1 out of every 5 American women past menopause is using estrogen replacement therapy, the incidence of breast cancer is 105 cases for every 100,000 women. There are an average 180,000 new cases a year; every year, more than 46,000 American women succumb to this terrible disease.

The evidence of a relationship between the increase in the exposure to estrogens and the increase in cases of breast cancer is clear for those who are willing to see it. At least thirteen major studies testify to a link between ERT and a higher risk of breast cancer among current or long-term users. Another eleven studies tie birth control pills to a similarly increased risk of breast cancer among women who use The Pill while they are very young or for long periods of time; the 1992 edition of *The Merck Manual* puts the danger point at more than four years' use prior to a first pregnancy.

But if the increase in breast tumors is due to an increased exposure to estrogen, The Pill and ERT aren't the only culprits. A life-style that exposes women to greater amounts of the estrogen secreted naturally by the body must also share part of the blame.

As Malcolm Pike proposes, one cause of the current breast cancer epidemic may well be our increased exposure to the estrogen produced naturally in our bodies. At a 1992 conference on cancer prevention in Boston sponsored by the General Motors Cancer Research Foundation and the Harvard School of Public Health, Pike explained that two hundred years ago the average woman did not have her first period until age seventeen, delivered and nursed as many as eight infants, and ovulated only 150 times in her entire lifetime. Her exposure to endogenous estrogen and her risk of breast cancer was dramatically lower than that of a modern American woman who is likely to start menstruating by the time she is twelve and go on to have only one or two children. As a result, she may ovulate as often as 450 times during forty years of fertility.

The notion that a woman's exposure to hormones produced naturally in her body can increase her risk of breast cancer is not new. In fact, you can trace it back three hundred years to the observations of an early Italian epidemiologist named Bernardino Ramazzini. In 1700, Ramazzini became the first to note an unusually high incidence of breast cancer among nuns. "You seldom find," he wrote, "a convent that does not harbor this accursed pest, cancer, within its walls."

A century and a half later, in 1842, another Italian scientist, this time a physician named Rigoni Stern, stood before a congress of his fellow surgeons to deliver an analysis of the cancer deaths in Verona, Italy. Like Ramazzini, Stern had found the highest incidence of breast cancer among the women least likely to become pregnant—nuns and unmarried women. Two years later, having reexamined his statistics, Stern concluded that breast cancer was also more common among older women.

With these three papers, Ramazzini and Rigoni Stern became the first persons to identify a natural risk factor for breast cancer: The continued exposure to endogenous estrogen resulting from a woman's failure to become pregnant. Today, it is widely accepted that early menarche and late menopause also increase a woman's exposure to estrogen throughout her reproductive years, thus raising her risk of breast cancer.

But exposure to endogenous estrogen is an *involuntary* risk factor. There is little or nothing a woman can do to change the genetic programming that makes her body work the way it does.

That is precisely why oral contraceptives and estrogen replacement therapy occupy a special place as risk factors in the present breast cancer epidemic: They are *voluntary* risks.

In the end, it comes down to this: No woman can turn off her ovaries at will. But any woman can refuse to take a pill.

# An Agenda for Women

# chapter 19

# Women's Rights, Women's Lives

## *A Blueprint for the Future*

Sir William Osler, the eminent nineteenth-century Canadian-born physician, said that the desire for medicine was "perhaps the greatest feature which distinguishes man from animals." Then, having credited patients with the sense to seek a cure, he warned doctors to hold up their end of the bargain: "Do not," he said, "pour strange medicines into your patients."

Osler died in 1919 at the age of seventy, ten years before the first estrogen was isolated and identified, but his commonsense observations perfectly describe the estrogen dilemma: Women who want its benefits and doctors who know its risks.

There is nothing new about our need to balance risk against benefits when using powerful medicine. Aspirin cures a headache but can make an ulcer bleed. Penicillin cures infection but can trigger a potentially fatal allergic reaction. Estrogen, which protects bones and heart, may either initiate a tumor or promote its growth.

Today, as the breast cancer epidemic rages around us, it is time to bring to estrogen the same caution we apply to literally dozens of other powerful drugs. No sensible person argues that estrogen should be banned, but no one suggests that it is safe for every woman.

We need to find a middle ground, one that protects women who might be harmed by birth control pills and hormone replacement therapy, while ensuring that women for whom these products pose a minimal risk, or no risk at all, are able to get the drug they want and need.

Here are seven ways to start:

1. *Tell the truth about estrogen.* Nearly a century has gone by since Glasgow surgeon Sir George Beatson published his account of breast tumors whose growth was slowed by removal of the patient's ovaries. It is thirty years since *The Merck Index* labeled estradiol a carcinogen linked to female reproductive tumors. It is twenty years since the AMA's Council on Drugs issued a statement acknowledging that estrogen, the once-mysterious "female principle," could make tumors grow.

In 1964, U.S. surgeon general Luther Terry galvanized the fight against lung cancer with the publication of the *Surgeon General's Report on Smoking and Health,* which documented the link between smoking and lung cancer. It is past time for the surgeon general and the FDA to shine the same bright light on estrogen products, to say out loud and in print what everyone knows to be true: Estrogen promotes the growth of existing tumors and may initiate cancers in susceptible women.

In February 1990, nearly ten months before the Nurses Health Study published its warning to current users of ERT, the FDA revised its labeling guidance for class information on noncontraceptive estrogen products to include the following paragraph:

While the majority of studies have not shown an increased risk of breast cancer in women who have ever used estrogen replacement therapy, some have reported a moderately increased risk (relative risks of 1.3–2.0) in those taking higher doses or those taking lower doses for prolonged periods of time, especially in excess of 10 years. Other studies have not shown this relationship.

This was a significant step forward in making information about estrogen and cancer available to doctors and patients. But rewriting the warnings is not the same as putting the information into women's hands. In the summer of 1992, CIBA Consumer Pharmaceuticals, the marketers of the transdermal estrogen patch Estraderm, submitted to the FDA a draft for new product information labeling that incorporated the 1991 FDA changes regarding breast cancer. In the fall of 1992 the company was still awaiting approval from the agency, with no firm idea of when it would arrive. As of the end of 1992, the FDA's new information about breast cancer and estrogen still does not appear in advertisements or package inserts for some post-menopausal estrogen products.

Clearly, we need to streamline the approval process for putting new information on drug package labels and in package inserts, so that we get new information out into the marketplace as quickly as possible after it appears in print.

And we need to enforce "truth in advertising" for estrogen products. In 1992, Ortho Pharmaceuticals released a new advertisement for its birth control pill, Ortho-Novum 7/7/7. The ads stress The Pill's ability to protect against ovarian and endometrial cancers and say that there is no overall increase in breast cancers among pill users. But as Cindy Pearson, program director of the National Women's Health Network, says, although "the words may be technically accurate, [they] are very misleading. By saying there is no overall increase in breast cancer Ortho is willfully hiding from women the fact that several studies have found a consistent increase in breast cancer among young women who took the pill for more than five years before becoming pregnant for the first time."

2. *Identify the women at risk.* In 1971, Edward Lewison wrote that it would be prudent for "women with a 'high-risk' predisposition for breast cancer and patients with known precursors of breast cancer [to] avoid the stimulation of long-term estrogen treatment and prevent the possibility of tumor progression. Whereas the individual sensitivity to hormonal stimulation may vary greatly from person to person and from age to age, yet in the matter of malignancy, it is wiser to be safe than sorry."

Today epidemiologists can draw the same rough outline of the women at risk that Lewison knew about in 1971: women who have close relatives with breast cancer, who begin to menstruate at a very early age, who reach menopause later than normal (the average age is currently fifty-two), who have their first full-term pregnancy after the age of thirty, or who have no children at all.

But these guidelines are old news, and worse yet, they do not predict real risk for real people. Delaying your first pregnancy until you are thirty or older may raise your risk of breast cancer, but no cancer expert can say with certainty that a woman who has her first child at thirty-two (or has no children at all) is fated to end up with breast cancer—or, conversely, that having a child at eighteen will guarantee she won't.

There is, however, new promise in the possibility that our increasing understanding of genetic activity may make it possible for us to find out who is truly at risk not just for breast cancer but for other kinds of cancer, too. In 1990, researchers at University of California, Berkeley, identified a region on one chromosome that appears to be strongly linked to early development of breast cancer. Women who inherit a defect in this region have a high risk of breast cancer before age forty-five, often in both breasts. This family form of breast cancer occurs in only 5 percent of all breast cancer patients, but some researchers now think that the genetic defect, the inherited susceptibility to various kinds of breast cancer, may be more common than previously thought.

We need a reliable test to screen for genetic defects that may put women at risk of breast cancer. Perfect that, and you make it possible to identify the women who need to pay special attention to early detection and who, not incidentally, should avoid estrogens. Developing such a test should be a high priority of the newly established National Institutes of Health Office of Research on Women's Health.

3. *Tighten the rules for prescribing estrogen.* When women using the original high-estrogen birth control pill developed blood clots and other serious side effects, some health advocates called for the FDA to take The Pill off the market. Today, the growing evidence of a link between pill use and an increased risk of breast cancer for some groups of women might prompt the same demand, but it was wrong then, and it would be wrong now.

"Even if future studies were to find that OCs were indeed related to [breast cancer]," says Susan Harlap, M.D., chief of the epidemiology service at Memorial Sloan-Kettering Cancer Center and one of the authors of the Guttmacher study, "that finding would have to be weighed against their benefit in averting other cancers." And, she adds, it must be weighed against the natural hazards of pregnancy, especially in undeveloped countries. "The news that oral contraceptives are dangerous filters down to India and Kenya and other undeveloped countries, where women believe The Pill will kill them," Harlap says. "But the truth is that women there are already dying of pregnancy."

In short, the real message of the new studies is not that we should abandon The Pill or ERT. It is that we should use them more judiciously.

Every drug has side effects: the surest path to a sleepless night is to read through the *Physicians' Desk Reference*. But there is virtually no side effect so horrendous that it will prevent a drug's being used if it is effective and if the situation warrants, for as Hippocrates is reported to have said: "For extreme illnesses, extreme treatments are most fitting."

So the point is to tailor the drug to the audience. Just as no reputable doctor would give penicillin to a patient who is allergic to it, no doctor should give estrogen to a woman whose history suggests that she may be exquisitely sensitive to its carcinogenic effects. For women with a family history of osteoporosis, the benefits of HRT may outweigh the risks. For women with a family history of breast cancer, the opposite may be true. Either way, the only responsible course is to reduce the indiscriminate prescription of estrogen products.

4. *Create a safer pill.* By 1975 most American women using The Pill were taking lower-estrogen products less likely to trigger blood clots and vascular disorders. But the choice of a high-estrogen pill remained a very real option until 1988 when the FDA formally ruled that no oral contraceptive should contain more than 50 mcg estrogen. Today, some researchers are looking at new ways to make oral contraceptives safer by manipulating the levels of female hormones in The Pill or by using other chemicals to prevent conception.

In March 1991, Dutch physician Michael Cohen unveiled his formula for a new pill he had tested on approximately a thousand women in Holland for four years without producing any side effects among the six hundred women who stayed through the entire trial. The pill contains progesterone and melatonin, a hormone secreted by the pineal gland, a small, pine-cone shaped body in the brain that helps regulate the monthly menstrual cycle. Together, progesterone and melatonin seem to prevent pregnancy as effectively as the estrogen/progestin pill, but Dr. Cohen speculates that unlike estrogen, melatonin stops the monthly buildup of specialized cells in the breast that will produce milk if a woman becomes pregnant. These cells often stay clumped together in the breast after ovulation even if conception does not occur, and Cohen thinks they may go on to become the nucleus of a breast tumor.

Malcolm Pike has suggested another possible solution based on how a woman's body behaves during the menstrual cycle. "We have known for ten years," he says, "that birth control pills significantly reduce the risk of cancers of the endometrium and ovaries. In the estrogen/progestin pill, the progestin is the dominant chemical. Cells in the ovaries also stop dividing because The Pill suppresses pituitary hormones that normally cause ovarian activity (and indirectly trigger ovarian cell division). This reduced endometrial and ovarian cell activity is the basis for claiming that The Pill protects against endometrial and ovarian cancers.

"The current birth control pill does not reduce the activity of cells in the breast because progestins do not slow down the reproduction of breast cells and estrogen stimulates it. However, if one were able to make an oral contraceptive with a significantly lower amount of both estrogen and progestin, use of such contraceptives might protect against breast cancer.

"The main problem with reducing the amount of estrogen and progestins is how to maintain The Pill's effectiveness as a method of birth control. One possibility is to add a third hormone, GnRH (gonadoptrophin-releasing hormone). GnRH is a natural hormone that controls the production of hormones in the ovary. GnRH agonists are synthetic hormones that interfere with the action of GnRH. Adding a GnRH agonist to suppress ovulation, while including just enough estrogen and progestin to maintain healthy bones and a healthy heart, might enable us to produce a contraceptive that prevents breast cancer." The National Institutes of Health should fund the studies needed to show whether these pills or some other innovative products are safer and more effective than the current pills.*

5. *Use hormone replacement therapy only when necessary.* All women lose bone density in the first five years after menopause; some lose considerably more than others. Good

---

*Two chemical contraceptives, Norplant and Depo-Provera, are estrogen-free but not free of problems. Norplant is a reversible, five-year contraceptive consisting of six thin capsules of levonorgestrel (a synthetic progestin) inserted under the skin of the upper arm. Twenty-four hours after the capsules are implanted under local anesthesia, the progestins begin to protect against conception. Norplant is an effective contraceptive, with some side effects such as bleeding irregularities and, extremely rarely, ectopic pregnancy (the pregnancy that occurs when a fertilized egg implants and begins to develop in the fallopian tube rather than the uterus). Its effects on breast cancer are unknown.

Depo-Provera, an injectible contraceptive, is a synthetic progesterone currently used in ninety countries around the world. Since 1972 it has been available in this country as a treatment for endometrial and kidney cancer. But in the early 1970s it was shown to cause breast tumors in beagle dogs and thus had never been approved for use as a contraceptive.

That changed in October 1992 when the FDA finally said yes to Depo-Provera. As of January 1993 it will be available as a contraceptive. This decision was applauded by Dr. Rosemary Thau, director of contraceptive development at the Population Council in New York, who called it a safe and effective means of birth control, and by David J. Andrews, acting director of Planned Parenthood Federation of America, who said the decision was "long overdue."

But the FDA warns that Depo-Provera is not for women who have liver disease, breast cancer, unexplained vaginal bleeding, or blood clots. Whether it will prove problematic for others remains to be seen. Even as an FDA panel was meeting to approve the new contraceptive, a WHO study showed a slightly increased rate of breast cancer—and a lower rate of endometrial cancer—among Depo-Provera users younger than thirty-five.

reasons to take hormones at menopause are: a high risk of osteoporosis (as demonstrated by a family history of the condition or a test that shows seriously reduced bone density) or a high risk of heart disease (again, a family history is the best indication). Good reasons to avoid hormones are: a family history of breast cancer; a personal history of breast cancer, endometrial cancer, vaginal bleeding, or liver disease.

Women who do not fit into either one of these obvious "yes" or "no" categories and wish to use estrogens to relieve hot flushes or any other menopausal discomfort should be thoroughly informed about the risks and benefits of estrogen; no doctor should prescribe estrogen without taking the patient's complete medical history or without discussing the nondrug alternatives to estrogens.

Drug companies prosper when women take estrogens and prosper again when these same women need drugs to cure the ills the hormones cause. They should be required by law to publicize the problems hormones may cause with the same energy they devote to advertising and promoting the value of post-menopausal replacement.

6. *Narrow the market for estrogens by promoting safe alternatives to chemical contraception and hormone replacement therapy.* In the United States, it is the unusual woman who is sexually active and decides never to use oral contraceptives. Some experts estimate that by the time they turn thirty-five, 80 percent of all young, sexually active American women will have used The Pill. Given the limited choice of contraceptive methods, says Cindy Pearson of the National Women's Health Network, "we would be almost hypocritical in describing ourselves as anti-Pill. But we think that our contraceptive research priorities have to be turned around so that we stop looking for a 'magic bullet,' the one drug–type contraceptive that will be 100 percent effective and free of side effects. We

ought to pour 90 percent of our research money into birth control methods that prevent sexually transmitted diseases, are easy to use, and are inoffensive to both men and women: viricides, new spermicides, new kinds of barrier methods for men and women. In 1992 there are signs that this may be happening, rumors even that the Population Council, the establishment's Mecca of all steroidal methods, is considering funding research on a viricide that a woman can apply in private and that will remain active for some time. We know it is a reaction to AIDS, but we would hope it will lead to providing women-controlled methods of contraception as well as protection against disease.''

As for post-menopausal hormone replacement, there are viable alternatives here, too. Contrary to earlier beliefs, new research suggests that a healthy diet, high in calcium, with adequate vitamin D (which helps get calcium into bones), continues to protect bones even among older persons. It is important to let women know that it is okay to eat enough food to maintain a healthy weight because when it comes to osteoporosis, the Duchess of Windsor's famous observation that a woman cannot be too rich or too thin was certainly half wrong. The frailer a woman is as she grows older, the more likely she is to end up with fractured bones. Regular exercise, which can include something as simple as a brisk half-hour walk every day, strengthens muscles (which cushion the bones) and may strengthen weight-bearing bones as well, although the evidence for this latter claim is still unclear.

7. *Tread carefully in the fields of preventive medicine.* Tamoxifen (Nolvadex) is a synthetic hormone whose chemical structure is similar to that of estrogen. It fights breast cancer by competing with estrogen for space on estrogen receptors in the tumor tissue. Every tamoxifen molecule that hooks onto an estrogen receptor prevents the linkage of an estrogen at the same site. Without a steady supply of estrogen,

cells in an estrogen receptor positive (ER+) tumor will not thrive and the tumor's ability to spread will be reduced.

Overall, taking tamoxifen seems to reduce the risk of death from a first tumor by about one-fifth and the risk of a recurrence by about 25 percent. Between 8 and 10 of every 100 breast cancer patients who get tamoxifen can expect to survive another ten years.

Now some experts are suggesting that tamoxifen may work in healthy women, preventing breast cancer from showing up in the first place. In 1991 the National Cancer Institute announced plans for a study to be conducted at 116 medical centers and 300 satellite institutions in the United States and Canada. The study will follow a group of 16,000 healthy, symptom-free women over thirty-five believed to be at high risk for breast cancer because they have one or more major risk factors such as early menarche, late first pregnancy (or no pregnancies at all), close female relatives with breast cancer, or a personal history of benign breast disease. For five years, half the women will take tamoxifen tablets, the other half a placebo. NCI will check the incidence of breast cancer at the five-year mark and, if the signs are favorable, will continue the study for another five years to see if taking tamoxifen lowers the expected incidence of breast cancer in this high-risk cohort.

For many women, the reaction to this has been one of expectant relief: At last, the government is doing something to protect us against breast cancer. Among some experts, however, the announcement set off a round of protests. "The tamoxifen trial is a perversion of prevention," said Adriane Fugh-Berman, M.D., of the Washington, D.C.–based National Women's Health Network. The problem, says Dr. Fugh-Berman, is that unlike other public health measures such as fluoridation of the water supply or the enrichment of milk with vitamin D, treatment with tamoxifen carries specific risks for healthy people.

About 25 percent of the women who take tamoxifen experience such "minor" side effects as hot flushes, fluid retention, and weight gain that can be controlled by reducing the dose. Other side effects may include nausea and vomiting; vaginal bleeding, itchiness, or discharge; skin rashes; alteration in the sensation of taste; depression; lightheadedness or headache; and cataract and retinal injuries. Tamoxifen has also been linked to the formation of blood clots in about 1 woman in 800 a year. When used to treat cancer, tamoxifen may make some tumors worse for a while, but this effect goes away quickly.

University of Pittsburgh breast cancer researcher Bernard Fisher, M.D., the principal investigator for the NCI study, contends that these adverse effects are rare and that they are unlikely to be so severe that a woman would have to stop using the drug. If the trial really works, he said in 1991, long-term use of tamoxifen by American women might prevent 36,000 invasive breast cancers and 34,000 heart attacks every year.

But now there are fears that tamoxifen, like estrogen, may be potentially carcinogenic.

In April 1992, a team of researchers at City Hospital in Nottingham, England, published a report in *Lancet* describing the death of a fifty-eight-year-old woman who had been taking 240 mg tamoxifen a day, the same dose proposed for the NCI trial. Five months into treatment, she became jaundiced, and although her doctor immediately stopped the tamoxifen, she died. When an autopsy was performed, the doctors found liver cell damage. In addition, her body's ability to produce the white blood cells that fight infection was suppressed.

Her doctors then began looking for reports of other women who had experienced problems with tamoxifen. They found that the U.K. Committee on Safety of Medicines knew of at least nine other cases in which tamoxifen had caused liver damage (four of them fatal), plus another eleven cases of nonfatal liver complications. There were no similar reports in the United States, but in 1989, oncologist Lars E. Rutqvist of Karolinska Institute in Stockholm, Sweden, reported two primary liver tumors among breast cancer patients in a randomized trial of tamoxifen, four times the expected incidence rate.* To date, no other investigators have come up with this result, but there is some question as to whether they actually looked for it or simply assumed that any liver tumors in breast cancer patients were mestastases. Rutqvist's studies also suggested that women using tamoxifen were more likely to develop gastrointestinal tumors.

In 1992, researchers at the University of Miami School of Medicine in Florida backed up Rutqvist's discovery with a study of their own. In this study, as in so many earlier ones, laboratory animals who were given tamoxifen along with a known carcinogen were less likely to develop breast cancer. But among the animals that did develop breast cancer, there was an unusually high number of hormone-independent breast tumors, a type of tumor considered very hard to treat because it does not respond to treatment with hormones. Among the tamoxifen-treated rats, hormone-independent tumors grew three times faster than they did in animals not taking tamoxifen.*

The British Medical Research Council (MRC) has with-

---

*How can two tumors be four times normal? Assume that the expected incidence of liver tumors is 1 for each 200 women. If the study includes only 100 women, the expected incidence would be (theoretically) ½ tumor. Thus, two tumors among these 100 women would be four times the expected rate.

*Taking tamoxifen may also increase the risk of endometrial cancer, a risk Richard Peto downgrades with the explanation: "Endometrial cancer caught early seldom kills ... [so] it's 'no big deal.' " This explanation infuriates many women, including Fugh-Berman, who notes that the treatment for endometrial cancer is hysterectomy. "To some of us," she says, "it's a big deal to lose your uterus."

drawn funding for additional tamoxifen studies because, as MRC secretary Dai A. Rees explained, nobody has established a dose level above which the drug is dangerous, which means it is impossible to find a dose presumed to be safe, a basic requirement for testing drugs on healthy people. *This caution does not apply to women who already have breast cancer and are being treated with tamoxifen. For these women, tamoxifen is still considered "a well-tried and effective treatment."*

While waiting for the British Department of Health to approve their trials, the Imperial Cancer Research Fund and the Cancer Research Campaign decided in April 1992 to continue on their own. Similar long-term studies are on the drawing boards in Europe and Australia, and the U.S. trials are, as this is written, about to begin. Right now, no one can say whether they will turn out to be a clear win for women or just another well-intentioned but ultimately destructive rerun of the estrogen dilemma.

## Confronting Reality

Throughout the 1980s, as the incidence of breast cancer in the United States continued to rise, American women and their doctors searched for reasonable explanations for the epidemic.

Some, however, denied there *was* an epidemic, choosing instead to attribute the increase in cancers solely to the increase in the number of older women.

Alas, this is the wrong answer. It, is as we have seen, untrue, which means it is an explanation no one will believe. What's more, to deny that we are contending with an epidemic is to instruct thousands of American women to relax and accept the inevitable.

In fact, there is a logical explanation for what is happening. It runs like a ribbon through all the research leading to known and suspected risk factors for breast cancer. The explanation begins with Ramazzini's finding a higher rate of breast cancer among Italian nuns. It continues with Beatson's discovery that removing a breast cancer patient's ovaries might slow the progress of her disease. It is drawn from the animal studies of the 1930s and 1940s, Malcolm Pike's data connecting The Pill to breast cancer in young women, Robert Hoover's Kentucky report of a link to ERT, and all the confirming studies since.

The explanation is this: Exposure to estrogen—both the estrogen produced in a woman's own body and the estrogen she takes in a variety of drugs—increases the risk of breast cancer.

To accept this is not to say that every woman who takes estrogen or whose lifestyle exposes her to larger amounts of naturally secreted estrogen will develop breast cancer, or that every woman who develops breast cancer will have experienced these risk factors.

But there is no longer any doubt that estrogen products are implicated in some cases of breast cancer. There is no doubt that diet and lifestyle count because women who are better fed live longer and are exposed to more naturally secreted estrogen.

In the end we must accept the evidence before our eyes without fear or prejudice. It is our only hope of defeating this terrible disease.

# Appendixes

Appendixes

# Estrogens and Breast Cancer: A Chronology

1929: The first estrogen (estrone) is isolated and identified

1931: First American woman given first injection of estrogen

1932: Estrogen injections produce malignant breast tumors in male laboratory mice

1934: First use of estrogens to treat symptoms of menopause

1937: Natural female hormones used to suppress ovulation in laboratory rabbits at Penn State University

*The incidence of breast cancer in the United States is 67 cases per 100,000 (white) women*

1938: Chemists at Schering Company produce estrogen pills

1940: The first oral estrogens for ERT go on sale

Scientists at the National Cancer Institute find synthetic estrogen diethylstilbestrol (DES) produces breast tumors in male and female laboratory mice

The leading causes of cancer deaths among American women are cancer of the uterus and cancer of stomach

The incidence of breast cancer in the United States is 59 cases for every 100,000 women

*An American woman's lifetime risk of breast cancer is 1-in-20*

1941: More than a dozen brands of estrogen are available for treatment of menopausal and menstrual disorders

Synthetic estrogen (DES) used to prevent miscarriage

1944: Syntex, a pharmaceutical company, created to manufacture and sell synthetic progesterone

1945: Cancer researchers discover that a chemical's ability to stimulate unregulated cell growth is one measure of its potential carcinogenicity

1950: The incidence of breast cancer in the United States is 65 cases for every 100,000 women

*An American woman's lifetime risk of breast cancer is 1-in-15*

1951: Birth control pioneer Margaret Sanger makes first donation to support Gregory Goodman Pincus' research on chemical contraceptives

Syntex steroid chemist Carl Djerassi patents nonethindrone, the first effective oral progestin

1952: More than thirty brands of estrogen products on the market: injectible solutions, pills, ointments, suppositories, and nasal sprays

1956: G.D. Searle and Planned Parenthood begin trials of the estrogen/progestin birth control pill in Puerto Rico

1957: FDA approves use of estrogen/progestin combination for medical conditions such as menstrual disorders

1960: FDA grants permission for Searle to market an estrogen/progestin product, Enovid-10, as an oral contraceptive

*The Merck Index* publishes its first warning of a link between estrogens and cancers of the breast and reproductive organs

*The incidence of breast cancer in the United States is 72 cases for every 100,000 women*

*An American woman's lifetime risk of breast cancer is now 1-in-14*

1961: 800,000 American women fill their first prescription for an oral contraceptive

1962: FDA approves a second oral contraceptive, Ortho Pharmaceuticals' Ortho-Novum

1963: 1.2 million American women are using The Pill

Robert Wilson meets "Mrs. P.G.," the woman whose use of Enovid-10 keeps her "young" at age fifty

1965: 1-in-4 married American women has used or is using birth control pills

1966: Robert Wilson publishes *Feminine Forever;* estimates that in 1967 the number of "sexually restored, post-menopausal women" will pass 14,000

1969: British Committee on Safety of Drugs recommends banning oral contraceptives containing more than 50 mcg estrogen

The First National Conference on Breast Cancer, sponsored by the American Cancer Society (ACS) and the U.S. Public Health Service, convenes in Washington, D.C.

*The ACS predicts 29,000 female breast cancer deaths*

*The incidence of breast cancer in the United States is 72.5 cases for every 10,000 white women; 60.1 cases for every 100,000 black women*

1970: First warning (blood clots) included in package insert for oral contraceptives

8.5 million American women are using birth control pills; 65 percent of them are "high-dose" products with more than 50 mcg estrogen

The American Medical Association's Council on Drugs says that estrogens may stimulate existing breast tumors to malignant activity

The incidence of breast cancer in the United States is 74 cases for every 100,000 women

*An American woman's lifetime risk of breast cancer is now 1-in-13*

1971: Synthetic estrogen (DES) reported to cause vaginal cancers in daughters of women who took the drug while pregnant

Second National Conference on Breast Cancer convenes in Los Angeles

1972: *Breast cancer is now the leading cause of cancer deaths among American women*

1973: 10 million American women, including 36 percent of all married women, are using birth control pills

1974: 70 percent of all married American woman have a "favorable view" of The Pill

5 million American women are using estrogens to relieve

menopausal symptoms

*The ACS predicts 90,000 new cases of female breast cancer and 33,000 deaths*

1975: An NCI study shows a six- to elevenfold increase in incidence of breast cancer among women with prior history of benign breast disease who had used The Pill for more than six years

Four separate studies show an increase as high as 50 percent in the incidence of endometrial cancer among women using estrogen products

1976: 22.3 percent of all fertile American women are using oral contraceptives

Approximately 6 million women are using ERT

Study of one doctor's practice in Kentucky shows an overall 30 percent increased risk of breast cancer among women using ERT

1977: *The incidence of breast cancer in the United States is 81 cases per 100,000 women*

1980: 19 percent of American women of childbearing age use The Pill

17 percent of all birth control pills sold in the United States still contain more than 50 mcg estrogen

A study in two Los Angeles retirement communities shows an 80 percent higher risk of breast cancer among women who take a cumulative lifetime dose of 1,500 mg estrogen

*The incidence of breast cancer in the United States is 90 cases for every 100,000 women*

*An American woman's lifetime risk of breast cancer is now 1-in-11*

1981: Researchers at the University of Southern California find a significant increase in the incidence of breast cancer among women who use oral contraceptives before a first full-term pregnancy

Researchers from the National Institutes of Health publish study of 1,600 women in twenty-nine cancer centers across the country showing that use of ERT may raise a woman's risk of breast cancer to nearly seven times higher than normal

1982: Following publicity about acute effects of oral contraceptives (blood clots, migraines, heart attack, stroke) the percentage of American married women using The Pill falls to 19.8

1983: 17 million prescriptions are written for estrogen

Second California study shows that women who use The Pill for more than four years before their first full-term pregnancy or before age twenty-five are four times more likely to develop breast cancer before age forty-five

1984: *New England Journal of Medicine* reports a 47 percent higher incidence of breast cancer among 4 million women who used DES while pregnant

*The ACS predicts 115,000 new cases of female breast cancer*

1985: 11.8 million American women age eighteen to forty-four are using The Pill, the leading reversible method of birth control in the United States; 25 percent of them are using it for longer than five years

1986: Nearly 12.5 million American women age fifteen to forty-four are using The Pill

FDA approves Estraderm, CIBA Pharmaceutical's new patch that delivers continual low doses of estrogen through the skin for post-menopausal ERT

*The ACS predicts 123,000 new cases of female breast cancer and 39,900 deaths*

1987: CASH study shows a more-than-200 percent increase in risk of breast cancer among fifty- to fifty-four-year-old women whose ovaries have been removed or who have a family history of breast cancer and who use ERT

*An American woman's lifetime risk of breast cancer is now 1-in-10*

1988: Approximately 14 million American women age fifteen to forty-four are using The Pill

Nineteen years after the British have acted, the FDA recommends removing from the market all oral contraceptives containing more than 50 mcg estrogen

*The ACS predicts 135,000 new cases of female breast cancer and 42,300 deaths*

1989: Nurses Health Study (121,000 married female nurses) show that women currently using oral contraceptives are 60 percent more likely than nonusers to develop breast cancer

3.5 million American women are using ERT

*The incidence of breast cancer in America is 105 cases per 100,000 women*

1990: 26 percent of American women of childbearing age are using The Pill

Nurses Health Study shows that women who use ERT are 30 to 40 percent more likely than nonusers to develop breast cancer

Incidence of ER+ tumors among American women is increasing five times faster than incidence of ER– tumors

*The ACS predicts 150,000 new cases of female breast cancer and 44,300 deaths*

1991: 16 million American women age fifteen to forty-four are using The Pill; 37 percent of them for five years or longer

15 percent of all post-menopausal American women are using ERT

A meta-analysis from the U.S. Centers for Disease Control attributes 4,708 new cases of breast cancer and 1,468 deaths a year to use of ERT

*An American woman's lifetime risk of breast cancer is now 1-in-9*

*The ACS predicts 175,000 new cases of female breast cancer and 44,500 deaths*

1992: *The National Cancer Institute predicts 180,000 new cases of female breast cancer and 46,000 deaths*

*An American woman's lifetime risk of breast cancer is now 1-in-8*

# Estrogens and Cancer: Studies That Show the Connection

*Table B-1.* **Estrogens and Endometrial Cancer**

| Date | Estrogen product | Study population (Authors) | Major conclusion |
|---|---|---|---|
| Oct 1975 | ERT | All females, San Francisco Bay area (California Tumor Registry) | 50 percent increase in cases, 1969–73, among older, affluent white women |
| Nov 1975 | OC | 27 women, age 21–37, from national registry of endometrial cancer patients (Silverberg/Makowski) | Uterine tumors linked to use of sequential birth control pills |
| Dec 1975 | ERT | Post-menopausal women at Kaiser-Permanente Health Plan (Ziel/Finkle) | Overall, risk 8 times higher w/ERT |
| Dec 1975 | OC | 117 endometrial cancer patients and controls, Washington State (Smith) | Overall, risk 4.5 times higher w/ERT |

OC = oral contraceptives
ERT = estrogen replacement therapy

*Table B-2.* **Estrogens and Breast Cancer**

| DATE | ESTROGEN PRODUCT | STUDY POPULATION (AUTHORS) | MAJOR CONCLUSION |
|------|------------------|----------------------------|------------------|
| Oct 1975 | OC | 898 women hospitalized in San Francisco w/breast cancer or breast disease; 872 healthy controls (Fasal/Paffenbarger) | 2–4 yrs' use OC = 90 percent higher risk |
| Aug 1976 | ERT | 1,891 women in one Kentucky doctor's practice (Hoover, et al.) | 5–9 yrs' use ERT = 20 percent higher risk; 10–14 yrs = 30 percent higher risk; 15 yrs = 100 percent higher risk |
| Apr 1980 | ERT | 178 patients under age 75 in 2 L.A. retirement communities (Ross, et al.) | 7 yrs' use ERT = 80 percent higher risk; cumulative dose/1,500 mg estrogen = 150 percent higher risk |
| Oct 1980 | OC | 16,638 women enrolled in Kaiser-Permanente Health Plan (Ramcharan/ Barendes) | Overall, no evidence of higher risk w/OC use; "slight excess risk," age 40–45 |
| Jan 1981 | OC | 163 L.A. breast cancer patients age 32 or less at diagnosis (Pike/Henderson) | Long-term OC use before age 25 = increased risk |
| May 1981 | ERT | 881 cases/865 controls from national breast cancer identification screening project (Hoover/Brinton) | Overall, 24 percent higher risk w/ERT; for women whose ovaries had been removed, ERT = 667 percent increase in risk |

| DATE | ESTROGEN PRODUCT | STUDY POPULATION (AUTHORS) | MAJOR CONCLUSION |
|---|---|---|---|
| Oct 1981 | ERT | 345 newly diagnosed patients at Kaiser-Permanente Health Plan (Hoover/Glass/ Finkle) | Overall, 40 percent higher risk w/ERT |
| 1983 | OC | 314 cases/314 controls age 37 or less at diagnosis (Pike/Henderson) | 8 yrs' use OC = 70 percent higher risk |
| Sept 1986 | OC | All reported cases in 1 yr in Sweden and Norway (Meirik) | 4–7 yrs' OC use = 20 percent higher risk; 8–11 yrs' = 40 percent higher risk; 11 yrs' = 220 percent higher risk |
| Jan 1987 | ERT | 1,369 cases/1,645 controls, CASH/SEER (Wingo) | Overall, no increase in risk; 200 percent increase in risk w/ERT for women age 50–54 w/family history of breast cancer |
| May 1989 | OC | British women patients younger than 36 (MacPhearson/ Pike/Vessey) | 4–8 yrs' OC use = 40 percent higher risk; 8 yrs+ = 74 percent higher risk |
| July 1989 | OC | Pre-menstrual women in Sweden (174 cases/459 controls) (Olsson, et al.) | OC use before age 20 = 480 percent higher risk; use before age 25 = 430 percent higher risk |

*Table B-2.* **Estrogens and Breast Cancer** *(cont.)*

| DATE | ESTROGEN PRODUCT | STUDY POPULATION (AUTHORS) | MAJOR CONCLUSION |
|------|------------------|---------------------------|------------------|
| Sept 1989 | OC | 118,273 women, Nurses Health Study (Willett, et al.) | Current use OC = 60 percent higher risk; at age 40–44, current use = 166 percent higher risk |
| Aug 1989 | ERT | 23,244 Swedish women (Bergkvist, Hoover, et al.) | Overall, 9 yrs' use ERT = 70 percent higher risk |
| Nov 1990 | ERT | 121,700 women, Nurses Health Study (Colditz, et al.) | Current use ERT = 40 percent higher risk |
| Mar | OC | American women, age 15–44 (Guttmacher Inst.) | Use of OC at age 25–44 = higher risk |
| Apr 1991 | ERT | CDC "meta-analysis" of 26 studies, 1976–89 | 15 yrs+ use ERT = 30 percent higher risk |
| June 1991 | OC | Cancer patients in 10 countries (WHO Collaborative Study) | Overall, current use OC = 66 percent higher risk |

OC = oral contraceptives
ERT = estrogen replacement therapy

# Notes

References that show only a name (or names) and date—
that is, Hertz 1969—refer to scientific papers whose titles are
listed in full in the bibliography.

Except where noted, all incidence and mortality statistics
are from the American Cancer Society.

## Introduction

page xv: Statistics on breast cancer from *Cancer in the United States:
Is there an epidemic?* New York: American Council on Science and
Health, June 1988, and "Lifetime Risk of Developing Breast
Cancer," American Cancer Society, 1991, *The New York Times*,
January 25, 1991; ibid., September 27, 1992.

## Part One    Estrogen

### 1. The Female Principle
page 3: Description of developing fetus: *The Columbia University
College of Physicians and Surgeons Complete Home Medical Guide*, rev.
ed. (New York: Crown Publishers, 1989), p. 202.
page 4: History and outlawing of castration: R. Brasch, *How Did
Sex Begin?* (New York: New American Library, 1974), p. 157.

page 5: Galen's discoveries, publication of Vesalius' book, Servetus' death, Church relents on dissection: Howard W. Haggard, M.D., *Devils, Drugs and Doctors* (New York: Harper & Row, 1929), pp. 130–47 *passim,* and Lois N. Magner, *A History of Medicine* (New York: Marcel Dekker, Inc., 1992) p. 191.

page 5: Introduction of anesthesia and antisepsis; Morton's operation and Warren's quote: ibid., p. 99–101. Semmelweis' problems in Vienna: Haggard, p. 87.

page 6: Lister's papers: ibid., p. 169. Use of wine, vinegar and chlorinated lime: Alfred Goodman Gilman, Louis S. Goodman, Alfred Gilman, *The Pharmacological Basis of Therapeutics*, 6th ed. (New York: Macmillan, 1980), p. 964.

page 7: Battey and "female castration," Currier: Janice Delaney, Mary Jane Lupton, Emily Toth, *The Curse* (New York: New American Library, 1977), p. 169. Beatson's report: cited in Hertz 1967, and Lewison 1971.

page 7: Emil Knauer's discovery: Goodman and Gilman, p. 1420.

page 8: Allen and Doisy's discovery: ibid.

page 8: Discovery of estrogen in blood, urine of sows, pregnant women: ibid.

page 8: Isolation of estrone: Hertz, 1967. Doisy's Nobel Prize: *World Almanac* (New York: World Almanac, 1991), p. 321.

page 9: Footnote on Pregnancy test: Goodman and Gilman, p. 1420, and Cathy Pinckney and Edward R. Pinckney, M.D., *The Patient's Guide to Medical Tests* (New York: Rawson Associates, 1977).

page 9: Body production of estrogen: Goodman and Gilman, p. 1420, and *The Merck Manual,* 15th ed. Rahway, N.J.: Merck Research Laboratories, 1987, p. 1687.

page 9: Daily production of estrogen: "Labeling Guidance for Non-contraceptive Drug Products, Physician Labeling," rev. 1990, U.S. Food and Drug Administration.

page 9: Metabolism of estrogen: Goodman and Gilman, pp. 1420–21.

page 11: Coronary Drug Project Research group: Goodman and Gilman, p. 1430, and Thomas J. Moore, *Heart Failure* (New York: Random House, 1989), p. 52.

page 11: Isolation of progesterone: *The Merck Index,* 11th ed. (Rahway, N.J.: Merck & Co., 1989), p. 1234. Testosterone: Goodman and Gilman, p. 1448. (This book was known as *Merck's Index* until the 5th ed. in 1940 when it was renamed *The Merck Index.)*

### 2. Menopause and Menstruation

page 13: Deutsch: cited in The Boston Women's Health Book Collective, *The New Our Bodies, Ourselves* (New York: Simon and Schuster, 1984), p. 444.

page 14: The "natural" menopause: Penny Wise Budoff, M.D., *No More Menstrual Cramps and Other Good News* (New York: G. P. Putnam's Sons, 1980), pp. 192–93.

page 14: Views of menopause from *Merck's Manual,* 4th ed. (New York: Merck & Co., 1911), p. 294; 5th ed. 1923, p. 178; *The Merck Manual,* 6th ed. 1934, p. 650; 7th ed. 1940, p. 590; 8th ed. 1950, p. 397; 13th ed. 1977, p. 912; 15th ed., 1987, p. 1713, 16th ed., 1992, p. 1793.

page 15: Use of ground bovine ovarian tissue: *Merck's Manual,* 1898, p. 54.

page 15: Hormones for menopause, first therapy: *Merck's Index,* 4th ed. (Rahway, N.J.: Merck & Co., 1930), p. 378. Cannabis: *The Merck Manual,* 6th ed., 1934, p. 6500.

page 15: Purified estrogen, "endocrine equilibrium," and messiness of injections: *The Merck Manual,* 7th ed. 1940, p. 592. Brands available in 1931: *The Merck Index,* 5th ed., 1940, p. 219. The first estrogen injection: Elizabeth Connell, *The Menopause Book* (New York: Hawthorne Books, 1977) p. 51.

page 16: Use of hormones for menstrual irregularities, *The Merck Manual,* 7th ed., 1940, p. 382, Lack of ovulation; ibid., p. 64.

page 16: Inhoffen's discovery: Carl Djerassi, *The Politics of Contraception* (New York: W. W. Norton, 1979), p. 247; and Willard Allen 1969. Creation of DES: Alfred Goodman Gilman, Louis S. Goodman, Alfred Gilman, *The Pharmacological Basis of Therapeutics,* 6th ed. (New York: Macmillan, 1980), p. 1422.

page 16: Drug laws: Steven Strauss and Max Sherman, "A Capsuled

History of Drug Law in the U.S.," *U.S. Pharmacist,* November 1985.

page 18: Footnote on number of women using estrogen: Robert A. Wilson, *Feminine Forever* (New York: David McKay, 1966), p. 21.

page 17: Course of treatment and side effects: *The Merck Manual,* 8th ed., 1950, p. 398; 9th ed., 1956, pp. 516–17.

page 18: Miscarriage, definition of: *The Merck Manual,* 15th ed., 1977, p. 1759. Statistics: The Boston Women's Health Collective, *The New Our Bodies, Ourselves* (New York: Simon and Schuster, 1984), p. 426.

page 18: The Smiths: Barbara Seaman and Gideon Seaman, M.D., *Women and the Crisis in Sex Hormones* (New York: Rawson Associates, 1977), p. 9.

page 19: Estrogens available in 1952: *The Merck Index,* 6th ed., 1952, pp. 401–2.

**3. Reproductive Remedies**

page 21: Sanger's quote: Paul Vaughn, *The Pill on Trial* (London: Weidenfeld and Nicolson, 1970), p. 25.

page 22: Pincus' research and his meeting with Sanger: ibid., pp. 28–29.

page 22: Research at Pennsylvania State University: John Rock, M.D., *The Time Has Come* (New York: Alfred Knopf, 1963), p. 162. Vaughn, p. 28.

page 22: Progesterone as "nature's contraceptive," Carl Djerassi, *The Politics of Contraception* (New York: W. W. Norton, 1979), p. 244.

page 24: Rock's early fertility studies and his philosophy: Rock. "Life mocks men's designs": ibid., p. 159. Natural hormones: ibid., pp. 162–63. Progesterone trials; ibid., pp. 163–64.

page 24: Need for large amounts of progesterone: Vaughn, pp. 30–31. Need for synthetic progestins: Rock, p. 162.

page 25: Marker's discovery of diosgenin: Vaughn, pp. 235–36. Formation of Syntex: ibid.

page 26: Djerassi, Hertz, patents on norethindrone: Vaughn, pp. 17–21. Disagreement with Searle: ibid., p. 31.

page 27: Pincus, Chang, Rock, the first hormones for contraception and infertility: Rock, pp. 164–65.

page 28: One scientist's warning in Tokyo: Vaughn, pp. 32–33.

page 28: Footnote on Baulieu and Pincus: *The New York Times,* January 26, 1992.

page 28: FDA approves progestins for menstrual disorders, Rock, p. 165 ff.

page 29: Drug testing regulations, Steven Strauss and Max Sherman, "A Capsulated History of Drug Law in the U.S., *U.S. Pharmacist,* November 1988.

page 30: Pincus and Chang's trials in Massachusetts, dosage: Vaughn, p. 32. Methods and results: ibid., pp. 37–38.

page 31: Choice of Puerto Rico: ibid., p. 39; Rock, p. 166.

page 31: Footnote: Gorton Carruth, *What Happened When,* New York: Harper & Row, 1989, pp. 349 and 368, and *The New York Times,* March 23, 1972.

page 31: Addition of estrogen to pill: Barbara Seaman and Gideon Seaman, *Women and the Crisis in Sex Hormones* (New York: Rawson Associates, 1977), p. 82.

page 32: Footnote on introduction of Norplant: "Wyeth-Ayerst Introduces Norplant System (levonorgestrel implants) an Alternative to Sterilization," New York: Lobsens-Stevens, press release, December 10, 1990.

page 32: Side effects of pill in Puerto Rico, Rock, p. 166, and Vaughn, pp. 47–48. Second Puerto Rican trial, Vaughn, pp. 47–48.

page 33: Deaths in Puerto Rico: Seaman and Seaman, p. 83.

page 33: FDA approval of birth control pill and number of women using it: *Twenty-third Annual Birth Control Study,* Ortho Pharmaceutical Corporation, 1991.

### 4. Problems with The Pill

page 35: Birth control pills as "adjuncts to nature": John Rock, *The Time Has Come* (New York: Alfred Knopf, 1963), p. 168.

page 36: British reaction: *The New York Times,* March 31, 1960. Pill approved in U.S.: *The New York Times,* May 10, 1960.

page 38: Blood clot deaths in California: *The New York Times,* September 7, 1969. FDA asks Searle to notify doctors: ibid., August 5, 1962. Number of women suffering side effects of The Pill, 1961–1962: ibid. Investigation by St. Louis coroner: ibid., August 7, 1962.

page 38: Calderone's defense, *The New York Times,* August 9, 1962.

page 38: Norway's ban of The Pill: *The New York Times,* August 7, 1962.

page 38: Footnote: Japan's ban: *The New York Times,* March 19, 1992.

page 39: Searle's concession to Larrick: *The New York Times,* August 7, 1962. Paniagua's defense of The Pill: ibid., August 18, 1962.

page 39: Crosson's denial: *The New York Times,* August 7, 1962.

page 39: Searle's Chicago conference, Barbara Seaman and Gideon Seaman, *Women and the Crisis in Sex Hormones* (New York: Rawson Associates, 1977), p. 85.

page 40: Searle's "golden egg": Paul Vaughn, *The Pill on Trial* (London: Weidenfeld and Nicolson, 1970), p. 49.

page 40: Quote from John G. Searle: ibid., p. 51.

page 41: Naming of the American Cancer Society: James T. Patterson, *The Dread Disease* (Cambridge, Mass.: Harvard University Press, 1987), pp. 71–72.

page 41: ACS failure to include estrogen as risk factor: "Cancer Facts & Figures 1991."

page 41: American Cancer Society supporters, and domination by medical establishment: Patterson, p. 72.

page 41: AMA's failure to find evidence of blood clots: *The New York Times,* August 10, 1962.

page 41: Footnote: Patterson, p. 117.

page 42: Connell's résumé: Seaman and Seaman, p. 102, and *The New York Times,* October 18, 1974.

page 42: American Cancer Society volunteers and relationship with NCI: Patterson, p. 169.

page 43: FDA report: *The New York Times,* September 7, 1969. Number of women using pill in 1963: Boston Women's Health

Collective, *The New Our Bodies, Ourselves* (New York: Simon & Schuster, 1984), p. 237. Number of women using ERT: Robert A. Wilson, *Feminine Forever* (New York: David McKay, 1966), p. 12.

### 5. Menopause Revisted

page 47: Wilson's credentials: Robert A. Wilson, *Feminine Forever* (New York: David McKay, 1966), title page. Wilson's views of menopause as a deficiency disease: ibid., p. 18. Wilson's meeting with "Mrs. P.G.": ibid., p. 78. Wilson's personal study, "Can a Woman Be Feminine Forever?," *The New Republic*, March 19, 1966. The "femininity index," and Wilson's hormone prescriptions: Robert A. Wilson, *Feminine Forever* (New York: David McKay, 1966) p. 116 ff, and Wilson, 1962.

page 48: "Women rich in estrogen": Wilson, p. 64. 100,000 copies: Barbara Seaman and Gideon Seaman, *Women and the Crisis in Sex Hormones* (New York: Rawson Associates, 1977), p. 350.

page 50: Hormone replacement theories: Wilson, 1962; *Look*, January 11, 1966; *Vogue*, June 1966. *The Medical Letter* is quoted in "Pills to Keep Woman Young," *Time*, April 1, 1966.

page 50: Wilson and the FDA: Seaman and Seaman, p. 353.

### 6. An Inference of Blame

page 51: FDA report: *The New York Times*, September 7, 1969.

page 52: Black's lawsuit; *The New York Times*, May 20 and 21, 1969. Buffalo lawsuit, against Searle: *The New York Times*, January 30, 1970.

page 52: Lasagna's quote: *The New York Times*, September 7, 1969.

page 52: FDA report: *The New York Times*, September 3, 1969, and September 7, 1969.

page 53: British report on low-dose birth control pills: *The New York Times*, April 24, 1970. U.S. delay: *The New York Times*, April 25, 1988.

page 54: Methodology of Puerto Rican study, Paul Vaughn, *The Pill on Trial* (London: Weidenfeld and Nicolson, 1970), pp. 44–47.

## Part Two Definitions, Statistics, and Studies

### 7. Defining the Disease

page 58: Definition of cancer: *The Columbia University College of Physicians and Surgeons Complete Home Medical Guide,* rev. ed. (New York: Crown Publishers, 1989), pp. 418–19.

page 58: Definition of breast cancers: *The Merck Manual,* 15th ed. (Rahway, N.J.: Merck Research Laboratories, 1987), pp. 1719–20.

page 59: Moskowitz quote: "The Muddle Over Screening Breast Cancer," *Medical World News,* May 9, 1988.

page 59: Footnote: "The Politics of Breast Cancer," *Newsweek,* December 10, 1990.

page 60: Incidence statistics: *Cancer in the United States: Is There an Epidemic?* New York: American Council on Science and Health, June 1988, and "180,000 New Cases of Breast Cancer," *U.S. Pharmacist,* February 1993.

### 8. Counting the Cases

page 62: Information on cancer rates before 1900: James T. Patterson, *The Dread Disease* (Cambridge, Mass.: Harvard University Press, 1987), pp. 31–32.

page 62: 1900 death rates: *Statistical Abstract of the United States, 1957* (Washington, D.C.: U.S. Government Printing Office, June 1957).

page 62: First statistics on cancer incidence: Feinlieb and Garrison 1969.

page 63: Introduction and updating of SEER: Bailar and Smith 1986.

page 64: Mammography as a confounding factor: ibid.

page 66: Increase in number of women over forty-four: *Information Please Almanac* (New York: McGraw-Hill, 1960), p. 525, and *World Almanac* (New York: World Almanac, 1991), p. 555.

### Part Three    Hormones and Cancer

*9. The Trail of Evidence*

page 71: Estrogen studies: Wynder and Schneiderman 1973.

page 72: Number of people required for an accurate study: Siegel and Corfman 1968.

page 72: Effects of endogeneous estrogen: Hertz 1967.

page 73: Estrogen as an anticarcinogen: Wilson 1962.

page 73: Ancient tests for poisons, Howard W. Haggard, *Devils, Drugs and Doctors* (New York: Harper & Row, 1929), p. 325.

page 74: Footnote on Ames test and DES: Carl Djerassi, *The Politics of Contraception* (New York: W. W. Norton, 1979), p. 53.

page 74: Lathrop and Loeb study: Lewison 1971.

page 75: Cell proliferation and carcinogenicity: Butterworth et al. 1991.

page 75: Lacassagne's experiments, Alfred Goodman Gilman, Louis S. Goodman, Alfred Gilman, *The Pharmacological Basis of Therapeutics*, 6th ed. (New York: Macmillan, 1980), p. 1445 and Lewison 1971.

page 75: Shimkin and Grady at NIH: Barbara Seaman and Gideon Seaman, *Women and the Crisis in Sex Hormones* (New York: Rawson Associates, 1977), p. 12.

page 75: Estrone as a carcinogen in laboratory rats: Ross 1980.

page 75: Wilson's dismissal of Lacassagne; Robert A. Wilson, *Feminine Forever* (New York: David McKay, 1966), p. 159.

page 75: The Smiths on Shimkin-Grady tests: Seaman and Seaman, p. 12.

page 76: Monkey studies: Hertz 1967. Wilson's comment: Wilson, p. 161

page 76: Djerassi on animal studies: Djerassi, pp. 53–54.

page 77: "Indirect evidence" of estrogen's carcinogenicity: Mac-Mahon and Cole 1969.

*10. Marking Time*

page 79: Hertz on the need to avoid unnecessary treatment with estrogens: *The New York Times*, October 23, 1963.

page 80: Estrogen responses in older versus younger women: Hertz 1967.

page 81: Hertz at First National Conference on Breast Cancer: Hertz 1969.

page 81: Bailar on estrogen safety: Bailar 1969.

page 82: The Nelson hearings, estrogens as "fertilizer": *The New York Times,* January 16, 1970. ACOG statement: *The New York Times,* January 18, 1970.

page 83: Gallup poll: *The New York Times,* February 2, 1970. Connell's statement: ibid., February 25, 1970. Pages of testimony: Carl Djerassi, *The Politics of Contraception* (New York: W. W. Norton, 1979), p. 93. New package insert: *The New York Times,* March 5, 1970.

page 83: AMA statement: Lewison 1971.

page 84: New procedures for testing contraceptive drugs, and WHO scientists: Djerassi, p. 57. Assessment of long-term risks and relationship of animal data to humans: ibid., pp. 53–54.

page 85: ACS estimates of incidence and deaths from breast cancer: *The New York Times,* May 18, 1971.

page 85: DES and vaginal cancers: *The New York Times,* May 2, 1971.

page 86: Report on Los Angeles conference: *The New York Times,* May 18, 1971.

page 87: Lewison's views on estrogen risks: Lewison 1971 and telephone interview with author, October 19, 1992.

page 87: Footnote: *The New York Times,* March 4, 1970.

### 11. First Reckoning

page 89: Number of women using birth control pills: *The New York Times,* February 2, 1970.

page 91: Gusberg report: Barbara Seaman and Gideon Seaman, *Women and the Crisis in Sex Hormones* (New York: Rawson Associates, 1977), pp. 349–50.

page 91: California Tumor Registry report: *The New York Times,* November 1, 1975, and editorial, *Journal of the American Medical Association (JAMA),* February 23, 1976.

page 92:  Sequential pills and cancer: *JAMA*, February 23, 1976, and Joe Graedon, *The People's Pharmacy* (New York: St. Martin's Press, 1977), p. 195. Brands and sales of sequentials: Graedon, p. 195, and Seaman and Seaman, pp. 96–97.

page 92:  Footnote on withdrawal of sequentials: *The New York Times*, February 26, 1976.

page 94:  Kaiser-Permanente study: *The New York Times*, December 18, 1975. University of Washington study: *JAMA*, February 23, 1976.

page 95:  Ayerst letter: Seaman and Seaman, p. 355.

page 96:  Walnut Creek Study: Ramcharan 1980. "The pill's vindication: how solid": *Medical World News*, November 24, 1980.

page 96:  Kaufman study: *Medical World News*, November 24, 1980.

page 96–97:  Comparison of studies on The Pill and reproductive cancers: Sidney M. Wolfe, M.D., *Women's Health Alert* (Reading, Mass.: Addison-Wesley, 1991), pp. 136–37.

page 97:  New ad for birth control pills: press kit from Ortho Pharmaceuticals, September 1992.

page 97:  Increase in risk for women using ERT: *Harrison's Principles of Internal Medicine*, 12th ed. (New York: McGraw Hill, 1991), p. 1793. Also, telephone interview with Wulf H. Utian, M.D., April 30, 1992.

page 98:  British report on male breast cancers: MacMahon and Cole 1969.

## *Part Four*  The Pill and Breast Cancer

### *12. An Important Warning*

page 101:  Rising incidence of breast cancer: *Cancer in the United States: Is There an Epidemic?*, New York: American Council on Science and Health, June 1988. Individual risks: "Lifetime Risk of Developing Breast Cancer," American Cancer Society, 1991. Breast cancer deaths: Fienlieb 1969.

page 102:  Paffenbarger résumé, telephone interview with author, September 21, 1992.

page 102:  San Francisco study of The Pill and breast cancer risk: Fasal and Paffenbarger 1975.

page 103: Women and breast cancer: James T. Patterson, *The Dread Disease* (Cambridge, Mass.: Harvard University Press, 1987), p. 13.

page 103: Strax: *The New York Times,* May 19, 1971.

page 104: History of mastectomy: Rose Kushner, *Breast Cancer* (New York: Harcourt Brace Jovanovich, 1975) p. 57.

page 104: Crile: *The New York Times,* May 20, 1971. Study on surgery for breast cancer: *The New York Times,* October 17, 1974.

page 105: Drug treatment: *The New York Times,* November 6, 1974 (L-PAM) and December 17, 1974 (Adriamycin).

page 106: Bayh quote: Marvella Bayh, with Mary Lynn Kotz, *A Personal Journey* (New York: Harcourt Brace Jovanovich, 1979), p. 222. Kushner, p. 107. FDA official on Ford and Rockefeller: *ibid.,* p. 126.

page 106: Footnote on DES: Kushner, p. 133 and *The New York Times,* September 10, 1975.

page 107: San Francisco study: Fasal and Paffenbarger 1975.

page 108: "An important warning": Hoover 1976, and telephone interview with author, September 8, 1992.

page 108: Follow-up conclusions: Paffenbarger and Fasal 1977.

page 108: Four studies: Romieu 1990.

page 110: Los Angeles study of young women: Pike 1981. Expansion of Los Angeles study: Pike 1983.

page 111: Favorable opinion of The Pill: Forrest and Henshaw 1983.

page 111: Incidence statistics: American Cancer Society, telephone interview, September 21, 1992.

### 13. The Official Truth

page 114: CDC epidemiologist: *The New York Times,* December 27, 1980.

page 115: CASH history: Sattin 1986.

page 115: First CASH study: "Pill exonerated in large study of breast cancer risk," *Medical World News,* December 20, 1982.

page 116: Stadel analysis: D. D. Edwards, "The Pill and Breast Cancer," *Science News,* November 9, 1985.

page 116: Cancer statistics: Wingo 1987. Wingo/Ory analysis: Sattin 1986.

page 117: "Generally reassuring": Schlesselman 1987.

### 14. Real Risk, Real Victims

page 120: Scandinavian data: Meirik 1986.

page 120: New Zealand study: Paul 1986.

page 120: Tyrer quote: Planned Parenthood Federation of America, Inc., memo to affiliate executive and medical directors, December 29, 1987.

page 121: Problems with the data: Wingo 1987.

page 121: New data from CASH: Sidney M. Wolfe, *Women's Health Alert* (Reading, Mass.: Addison-Wesley, 1991), p. 133.

page 122: Information about British women and The Pill: Chilvers 1989, and *The New York Times,* May 6, 1989.

page 122: Swedish premenopausal breast cancer patients: Olsson 1989.

page 123: Lack of information on CASH process: Graham Colditz, personal correspondence, September 1992.

page 124: Hoover quote: telephone interview with author.

page 125: The Nurses Health Study, Romieu 1989, and *The New York Times,* September 6, 1989.

page 126: Hormones to treat breast cancer: *The New York Times,* December 19, 1946.

page 126: Murphy quote: telephone interview with author, 1991.

page 126: Statistics on ER+ tumors: *The Merck Manual,* 15th ed. (Rahway, N.J.: Merck Research Laboratories, 1987), p. 1721. Modern use of androgens: ibid.

page 127: Kaiser-Permanente study on ER+ tumors: Glass 1990.

page 127: Hoover quote: telephone interview with author.

page 127: WHO study: Thomas 1991.

page 129: CDC meta-analysis: Steinberg 1991. Guttmacher study: Harlap, Kost, Forrest 1991. "Safe Sex, Safe Contraception": *The New York Times,* April 27, 1991.

page 130: Colditz comment: personal correspondence, September 1992.

page 131: Number of women using birth control pills: Press kit from Ortho Pharmaceuticals, September 1992.

## Part Five   ERT and Breast Cancer

### 15. No Protection

page 137: Wilson on hormones and reproductive cancers: Robert A. Wilson, *Feminine Forever* (New York: David McKay, 1966), p. 64.

page 137: New Jersey lawsuit: *The New York Times*, May 24, 1975.

page 138: Hoover's testimony: *The New York Times*, January 22, 1976; Barbara Seaman and Gideon Seaman. *Women and the Crisis in Sex Hormones* (New York: Rawson Associates, 1977), p. 410. Quote: telephone interview with author, September 8, 1992.

page 138: MacMahon's comments: telephone interview with author, September 9, 1992.

page 139: Hoover's Kentucky study: *The New York Times*, August 17, 1976, and Hoover 1976.

page 141: Scientists' quest for significant results: Victor Cohn, *News & Numbers* (Ames, Iowa: Iowa State University Press, 1989), p. 18.

page 142: Cancer statistics: *The New York Times*, March 27, 1975.

page 143: NIH report: "Estrogen Use and Postmenopausal Women," NIH Consensus Development Conference Summary, vol. 2, number 8. Washington, D.C.: National Institute on Aging, September 13–14, 1979.

page 144: Lilly settlement: *The New York Times*, January 19, 1980. California decision: *The New York Times*, March 21, 1980. U.S. Supreme Court action: *The New York Times*, October 15, 1980. New York Appeals Court action: *The New York Times*, February 25, 1981.

page 144: Breast cancer risk among DES mothers: Paul Kuehn, *Breast Cancer Care Options for the 1990s* (South Windsor, Conn.: Newmark Publishing, 1991), p. 65. Footnote: ibid.

page 144: Number of studies regarding ERT and breast cancer: Steinberg 1991.

page 145: Older women and ERT: Ross 1980.

page 145: Increases in risk: Brinton and Hoover 1981.

page 146: Increase in risk among peri-menopausal women on ERT: Hoover, Glass, Finkle, 1981.

page 146: Additional studies: Steinberg 1991.

page 147: Davis' cancer: Barbara Leaming, *Bette Davis* (New York: Simon and Schuster, 1992), pp. 328–30 *passim.*

page 147: Ireland on mastectomy: Jill Ireland, *Life Wish* (Boston: Little, Brown, 1987), p. 31.

page 148: Los Angeles conference, Crile, Crile, Urban, and Holleb: *The New York Times,* May 20, 1971. American Cancer Society meeting: *The New York Times,* October 17, 1974.

page 148: Vindication: *The New York Times,* March 14, 1985.

page 148: Reagan statement: Nancy Reagan with William Novak, *My Turn* (New York: Dell Publishing, 1990), p. 299.

page 149: Statistical decline in cases: *New York Newsday,* October 22, 1992.


### 16. Confirming Evidence

page 152: Swedish study: Bergkvist 1989, and *The New York Times,* August 3, 1989.

page 153: The effects of progestins and various estrogens: Barret-Connor 1989.

page 153: Estradiol and conjugated estrogens: *Merck's Index,* 11th ed. (Rahway, N.J.: Merck & Co., 1989), pp. 392, 583.

page 154: Brinton, Henderson, Pike: *The New York Times,* August 3, 1989.

page 155: Nurses Health Study: Colditz 1990; additional material from Colditz, telephone interview with author, 1991.

page 155: Brinton and Henderson: *The New York Times,* November 29, 1990.

page 156: American Cancer Society study: Garfinkel 1988. CDC study: Chu 1989. "The Politics of breast cancer," *Newsweek,* December 10, 1990.

page 156: Colditz: telephone interview with author, 1991. Heath quote: telephone interview with author, 1991.

page 156: Wilson statistics: Robert A. Wilson, *Feminine Forever* (New York: David McKay, 1966), p. 15, 21.

page 157: Meta-analysis: Steinberg 1991.

page 158: 3.5 million: M. Wolfe, *Women's Health Alert* (Reading, Mass.: Addison-Wesley, 1991) p. 95.

### 17. Defending ERT

page 160: Albright: Mary Ann Dunkin, "Estrogen replacement therapy," *Arthritis Today*, March-April 1991.

page 160: Estrogen and bone: *Harrison's Principles of Internal Medicine*, 12th ed. (New York: McGraw-Hill, 1991) p. 1921.

page 160: Nachtigall study: Penny Wise Budoff, *No More Menstrual Cramps and Other Good News* (New York: Penguin Books, 1981), p. 210.

page 160: Statistics on bone fractures: Sidney M. Wolfe, *Women's Health Alert* (Reading, Mass.: Addison-Wesley, 1991), p. 206.

page 161: NIH advice: *Osteoporosis*, National Institutes of Health, Consensus Development Conference Statement, volume 5, number 3, 1984.

page 162: Birnbaum quote: *The Washington Post*, May 8, 1985.

page 162: Estrogen approved for osteoporosis: *FDA Consumer*, April 1991. Estraderm introduced: *The New York Times*, September 17, 1986.

page 162: Statistics on heart disease: *1992 Heart and Stroke Facts* (Dallas, Tex.: American Heart Association, 1992).

page 162: British study: editorial, *JAMA*, February 23, 1976.

page 163: 1985 Nurses Health Study versus Framingham study: Stampfer 1991.

page 163: Footnote: Thomas J. Moore, *Heart Failure* (New York: Random House, 1989), pp. 33–34.

page 163: Two reports in Orlando: *Medical Weekly*, May 6, 1991.

page 164: New data from Nurses Health Study: Stampfer 1991. Statistics on death from heart attack versus death from breast cancer versus death from hip fracture: Goldman 1991.

page 164: Lack of random choice in nurses study: "Heart Benefits Found for Estrogen Users," *Science News*, September 14, 1991.

page 165: Goldman conclusion on ERT and heart disease and Gotto statement: *The New York Times*, September 12, 1991.

page 166: Dietary iron and the risk of heart attack: K. S. Fackelmann, "Excess Iron Linked to Heart Disease," *Science News*, September 19, 1992.

### 18. The Fatal Connection

page 167: Statistics on pill use: Press kit from Ortho Pharmaceuticals, 1992. Statistics on breast cancer incidence: American Cancer Society *Cancer Facts & Figures 1991*, and *U. S. Pharmacist*, February 1993. Individual risk: "Lifetime Risk of Developing Breast Cancer," American Cancer Society, 1991. Statistics on ERT use: *The New York Times*, September 16, 1991.

page 168: Use of birth control pills before pregnancy: *The Merck Manual*, 16th ed. (Rahway, N.J.: Merck Research Laboratories, 1992), p. 1816.

page 168: Pike: Kathy A. Fackelmann, "Motherhood and Cancer," *Science News*, October 31, 1992.

page 168: Ramazzini: James T. Patterson, *The Dread Disease* (Cambridge, Mass.: Harvard University Press, 1987), p. 13.

page 169: Rigoni Stern: Feinlieb 1969.

## Part Six   An Agenda for Women

### 19. Women's Rights, Women's Lives

page 173: Osler on desire to take medicine: Lewison 1971. "Strange medicine": Anthony Smith, *The Body* (New York: Viking, 1986), p. 527.

page 175: *Labeling guidance for estrogen drug products, physician labeling*, rev. February 1990, FDA.

page 175: CIBA product insert: telephone interview, CIBA, June 19, 1992.

page 176: Ortho 7/7/7: press kit from Ortho Pharmaceuticals, September 1992. Pearson quote: telephone interview with author, September 18, 1992.

page 176: "Wiser to be safe than sorry": Lewison 1971.

page 177: Researchers at University of California: Natalie Angier, "Gene That Checks Cell Growth May Be Key to Many Cancers," *The New York Times*, April 23, 1991.

page 177: Harlap quote: telephone interview with author, September 8, 1992. Hippocrates: John Bartlett, *Familiar Quotations*, 14th ed., ed. Emily Morrison Black (Boston: Little, Brown, 1968), p. 88.

page 179: Cohen's proposal: "Searching for a Better Pill," *Newsweek*, April 8, 1991.

page 180: Malcolm's Pike's proposal: telephone interview with author, August 14, 1992, and Spicer 1991

page 180: Footnote on Norplant: *Physician's Desk Reference*, 46th ed. (Montvale, N.J.: Medical Economics Data, 1992), pp. 2484ff.; Depo-Provera, "A New Birth-Control Option?," *Newsweek*, June 29, 1992.

page 182: Percentage of women using birth control pills: Pearson telephone interview with author. Calcium update: *Dairy Update*, National Dairy Board, October 1990.

page 183: Tamoxifen's benefit for eight to ten of every 100 women: Dana Points and Carla Rohlfing, "Breast Cancer Bulletin," *Family Circle*, April 1, 1992.

page 183: Scope of tamoxifen trial: Janet Raloff, "Tamoxifen Trial Begins Among New Cancers," *Science News*, May 9, 1992. Methodology of trial: *The New York Times*, October 23, 1992.

page 183: Fugh-Berman quote: Nancy Wartik, "Preventing Breast Cancer," *American Health*, September 1991.

page 184: Tamoxifen side effects: *The New York Times*, October 23, 1992; Raloff.

page 184: Fisher quote: Raloff.

page 185: Footnote, ibid.

page 184–85: British, Scandanavian, and Florida studies: ibid.

page 186: Conclusion that there is no epidemic: *The New York Times*, February 28, 1993.

# Bibliography

Note: Books and articles from the consumer press have been identified in full in the footnote section. The following bibliography lists studies published in professional journals.

Allen, Willard. Possible hazards in estrogen administration. *Cancer,* December 1969.

Bailer, John C., and Elaine M. Smith. Progress against cancer? *New England Journal of Medicine,* May 8, 1986.

Barrett-Connor, Elizabeth. Postmenopausal estrogen replacement and breast cancer (editorial). *New England Journal of Medicine,* August 3, 1989.

Bergkvist, Leif. The risk of breast cancer after estrogen and estrogen-progestin replacement. *New England Journal of Medicine,* August 3, 1989.

Boice, John D., Jr., and Richard R. Monson. Breast Cancer in women after repeated fluoroscopic examinations of the chest. *Journal of the National Cancer Institute,* September 1977.

Brinton, Louise A., Robert Hoover, et al. Menopausal estrogen use and risk of breast cancer. *Cancer,* May 15, 1981.

Bruzzi, P., et al., Short-term increase in risk of breast cancer after full-term pregnancy. *British Medical Journal,* 1988, 297:1096.

Butterworth, Byron E., Thomas L. Goldsworthy, James A. Popp, and Roger O. McClellan. The rodent cancer test: An assay under siege. CIIT Activities, Chemical Industry Institute of Toxicology, September 1991.

Chilvers, Clair, et al. Oral contraceptives and breast cancer risk in young women. *Lancet,* May 6, 1989.

Chu, Susan, et al. Alcohol consumption and the risk of breast cancer. *American Journal of Epidemiology,* 1989, vol. 130, no. 5.

Cohen, Leonard. Fiber and breast cancer. American Health Foundation, April 3, 1991.

Colditz, Graham A., et al. Prospective study of estrogen replacement therapy and risk of breast cancer in postmenopausal women. *Journal of the American Medical Association,* November 28, 1990.

Egan, R., et al. Report and commentary: The carcinogenic hazards of radiation to the breasts. *Cancer,* 1970, vol. 20, no. 24.

Fasal, Elfriede, and Ralph S. Paffenbarger. OC as related to cancer and benign lesions of breast. *Journal of the National Cancer Institute,* October 1975.

Fechner, R. E., Breast cancer during oc therapy. *Cancer,* December 1970, vol. 29.

Feinlieb, Manning, and Robert J. Garrison. Interpretation of the vital statistics of breast cancer. *Cancer,* December 1969.

Garfinkel, Lawrence, et al. NCI study: Alcohol and breast cancer, 1988.

Glass, Andrew, and Robert Hoover. Rising incidence of breast cancer: Relationship to stage and receptor status. *Journal of the National Cancer Institute,* April 18, 1990.

Goldman, Lee, and Anna N.A. Tostegon. Uncertainty about postmenopausal estrogen. *New England Journal of Medicine,* September 12, 1991.

Harlap, Susan. Oral contraceptives and breast cancer, cause and effect? *Journal of Reproductive Medicine,* May 1991.

Harlap, Susan, Kathryn Kost, Jacqueline Darroch Forrest. Preventing pregnancy, protecting health: A new look at birth control choices in the United States. New York: The Alan Guttmacher Institute, 1991.

Hertz, Roy. The problem of possible effects of oral contraceptives on cancer of the breast. *Cancer,* December 1969.

————. The role of steroid hormones in etiology and pathology of cancer. *American Journal of Obstetrics and Gynecology,* August 1, 1967.

Hildreth, Nancy G. The risk of breast cancer after irradiation of the thymus in infancy. *New England Journal of Medicine,* November 9, 1989.

Hoover, Robert, Andrew Glass, William D. Finkle, et al. Conjugated estrogens and breast cancer risk in women. *Journal of the National Cancer Institute,* October 1981.

Hoover, Robert, et al. Menopausal estrogens and breast cancer. *New England Journal of Medicine,* August 17, 1976.

Hulka, Barbara. When is the evidence for "no association" sufficient (editorial). *Journal of the American Medical Association,* July 6, 1984.

Hunter, David J., Talk to Society for Epidemiological Research in Buffalo, June 18, 1991.

Kaufman, David W., et al. Noncontraceptive estrogen use and the risk of breast cancer. *Journal of the American Medical Association,* July 6, 1984.

Kost, Kathryn, et al. Comparing the health risks and benefits of contraceptive choices. *Family Planning Perspectives,* March/April 1991.

Lewison, E. F., The Pill, estrogen, and the breast. *Cancer,* December 1971.

MacMahon, Brian, and Philip Cole. Endocrinology and epidemiology of breast cancer. *Cancer,* December 1969.

Matanoski, Genevieve M., et al. Electromagnetic field exposure and male breast cancer (letter). *Lancet,* March 23, 1991.

McGregor, D. H., et al. Breast cancer incidence among atomic bomb survivors at Hiroshima and Nagasaki, 1950-1969. *Journal of the National Cancer Institute,* September 1977.

Meirik, Olav, et al. Oral contraceptive use and breast cancer in young women: A joint national case/control study in Sweden and Norway. *Lancet,* September 20, 1986.

More critics raise voices against estrogen therapy. *Journal of the American Medical Association,* February 23, 1976.

Olsson, Hakan, et al. Early oc use and breast cancer among pre-menopausal women: Final report from a study in southern Sweden. *Journal of the National Cancer Institute,* July 5, 1989.

Paffenbarger, Ralph S., Elfriede Fasal, et al. Cancer risk as related to use of oral contraceptives during fertile years. *Cancer,* April supplement, 1977.

Paul, C., et al. Oral contraceptives and breast cancer, a national study. *British Medical Journal,* 1986, vol. 293.

Pike, M. C., et al. Oral contraceptive use and early abortion as risk factors for breast cancer in young women. *British Journal of Cancer,* 1981, vol. 43.

————. Breast cancer in young women and use of oral contraceptives: Possible modifying effect of formulation and age at use. *Lancet,* October 22, 1983.

————. Breast cancer and oral contraceptives. *Lancet,* November 23, 1985.

Ramcharan, Savitri, et al. The Walnut Creek contraceptive drug study. *Journal of Reproductive Medicine,* December (supplement), 1980.

Romieu, Isabelle, Jesse A. Berline, and Graham Colditz. Oral contraceptives and breast cancer. *Cancer,* December 1, 1990.

Romieu, Isabelle, Walter Willett, et al. Prospective study of oral contraceptive use and risk of breast cancer in women. *Journal of the National Cancer Institute,* September 6, 1989.

Rosenblatt, Karin A., et al. Breast cancer in men: Aspects of familial aggregation. *Journal of the National Cancer Institute,* June 19, 1991.

Ross, Ronald K., et al. A case-control study of menopause estrogen therapy and breast cancer. *Journal of the American Medical Association,* April 26, 1980.

Ross, William L., The magnitude of the breast cancer problem in the U.S.A. *Cancer,* December 1969.

Sattin, Richard W., et al. Oral contraceptive use and the risk of breast cancer. The Centers for Disease Control and National Institute of Child Health and Human Development Cancer and Steroid Hormone Study. *New England Journal of Medicine,* August 14, 1986.

Schlesselman, James J., Bruce V. Stadel, Pamela Murray, and

Sheng-han Lai. Breast cancer risk in relation to type of estrogen contained in oral contraceptives. *Contraception,* December 1987.

———. Breast cancer in relation to early use of oral contraceptives. *Journal of the American Medical Association,* March 1988.

Scott, Wendell G. Interdisciplinary approach to the control of cancer of the breast. *Cancer,* December 1969.

Shore, Roy E., et al. Breast neoplasms in women treated with X-rays for acute postpartum mastitis. *Journal of the National Cancer Institute,* September 1977.

Siegel, Daniel, and Philip Corfman. Epidemiological problems associated with studies of the safety of oral contraceptives. *Journal of the American Medical Association,* March 11, 1968.

Skegg, David C. G., Potential for bias in case-control studies of oral contraceptives and breast cancer. *American Journal of Epidemiology,* February 1988.

Spicer, Darcy V., Donna Shoupe, and Malcolm C. Pike. GrNH agonists as contraceptive agents: Predicted significantly reduced risk of breast cancer. *Contraception,* September 1991.

Stadel, Bruce V., and James J. Schlesselman. Oral contraceptive use and the risk of breast cancer in women with a prior history of benign breast disease. *American Journal of Epidemiology,* March 1986.

Stampfer, Meir J., Graham Colditz, et al. Post-menopausal estrogen therapy and cardiovascular disease. *New England Journal of Medicine,* September 12, 1991.

Steinberg, Karen K., et al. A meta-analysis of the effect of estrogen replacement therapy on the risk of breast cancer. *Journal of the American Medical Association,* April 17, 1991.

Thomas, D. B. The WHO collaborative study of neoplasia and steroid contraceptives: The influence of combined oral contraceptives on risk of neoplasms in developing and developed countries. *Contraception,* June 1991.

Vanderbroucke, Jan P. Postmenopausal estrogen and cardioprotection. *Lancet,* April 6, 1991 (follow-up letters, May 11, 1991).

Willett, Walter. Alcohol and breast cancer. *New England Journal of Medicine,* 1987, vol. 316, pp. 1174–80.

Willett, Walter, et al. Relation of meat, fat and fiber intake to the risk of colon cancer in a prospective study among women. *New England Journal of Medicine,* December 13, 1990.

Wilson, Robert A. The roles of estrogen and progesterone in breast and genital cancer. *Journal of the American Medical Association,* October 27, 1962.

Wingo, Phyllis, et al. The risk of breast cancer in post-menopausal women who have estrogen replacement therapy. *Journal of the American Medical Association,* January 9, 1987.

————. Eight specific differences in the relationship between oral contraceptive use and breast cancer. Conference on oral contraceptive and breast cancer, Irvine, California, 1990.

Wynder, Ernest L., and Marvin A. Schneiderman. Exogenous hormones—boon or culprit? (editorial). *Journal of the National Cancer Institute,* September 1973.

# Index

Abbott Laboratories, 143
Abortion, 21
  spontaneous, 18
ACS, 116, 126, 147, 155, 156
Adrenal glands, 9
Adriamycin, 105
AIDS, 38$n$, 61, 129, 182
Albright, Fuller, 160
Alcohol, 155–56
Allen, Edgar, 8, 74
American Cancer Society (ACS),
  41, 42, 64, 65, 77, 79, 85,
  90
American Chemical Society, 25
American College of Obstetri-
  cians and Gynecologists, 82,
  83
American College of Surgeons,
  41, 126
*American Journal of Obstetrics and
  Gynecology,* 91
American Medical Association
  (AMA), 41, 174
  Council on Drugs, 83, 86
Ames, Bruce N., 74$n$
Andrews, David, J., 180$n$
Androgens, 9
Anesthesia, 5, 104

Animal studies, 7, 8, 26–28, 31,
  73–78, 80, 82–84, 138, 142,
  185
Antiseptics, 6
Aschheim-Z pregnancy test, 8$n$
Austin, Donald F., 91, 93
Ayerst Laboratories, 50, 95

Bailar, John C., III, 81
Barrett-Connor, Elizabeth,
  152–54
Battey, Robert, 6
Baulieu, Etienne-Emile, 28$n$
Baxter, Anne, 147
Bayh, Marvella, 105
Beatson, George, 7, 74, 174,
  186–87
Bergkvist, Leif, 151–53, 155, 157
Birnbaum, Davi, 161–62
Birth control pills, 77–78, 159
  blood clots caused by, 37–39,
    41, 42, 51–53, 81–83, 86, 95,
    162, 177
  breast cancer and, 79, 80, 83–
    87, 90, 98, 101–2, 106–10,
    114–17, 119–25, 127–33,
    137, 138, 142, 146, 151, 154,

Birth control pills (*cont.*)
157, 167–69, 174–76, 179–
80, 187
concerns about long-term
safety of, 79–81
defense of, 40–42
development of, 21–22, 25–28
duration of use of, 76–77
endometrial cancer and, 91,
96
failure of FDA to act on,
52–54
heart disease and, 162
menopause and, 46–47, 50
package insert for, 83
popularity of, 89
safe alternatives to, 181–82
safer, 178–80
Senate hearings on, 79, 81–83
side effects of, 32–33, 35–37,
42, 52, 73
testing of, 28–33, 35, 53–54,
64–65, 83–84
tightening of rules for prescribing, 177–78
Black, Elizabeth, 51
Black, Raymond, 51, 81
Black, Shirley Temple, 105
Blood clots, 37–39, 41, 42, 51–
53, 81–83, 86, 95, 162,
177
Body fat, estrogen production
in, 9
Bone loss, 160–62, 180, 182
Bork, Robert, 31$n$
Boston University School of
Medicine, 163
Breast cancer, 58–60
age of onset of, 109–10, 121–
22, 130, 131, 133
alcohol consumption and,
155–56
animal research on, 74–77, 84,
98
annual number of deaths
from, 113–14, 142
attitudes toward, 103, 105

birth control pills and, 79, 80,
83–87, 90, 98, 101–2, 106–
10, 114–17, 119–25, 127–33,
137, 138, 142, 146, 151, 154,
157, 167–69, 174–76, 179–
80, 187
DES and, 144
epidemiology of, 64–68, 107
ERT and, 86, 90, 127, 137–46,
151–59, 164, 167–69, 174,
181, 187
estrogen receptor-positive
(ER+), 126–27, 183
identification of women at risk
for, 176–77
incidence of, 60, 68, 78, 93,
111, 113, 130, 139, 142,
148–49, 167, 186
ovariectomy in treatment of,
7, 72, 74, 77, 126, 187
prevention of, 182–86
retrospective studies of, 71–73
risk factors for, 41, 59, 90
treatment of, 103–5, 146–48
Breast Cancer Advisory Center,
148
Brevicon, 26$n$
Brigham and Women's Hospital
(Boston), 124
Brinton, Louise, 145, 154, 155
British Family Planning Association, 35
British Institute of Cancer Research, 121
*British Medical Journal*, 98
British Medical Research Council, 185–86
Brody, Jane E., 86
Budoff, Penny Wise, 13–14

Calderone, Mary S., 38
California, University of, Berke-
ley, 176
California State Dept. of Health,
Bureau of Chronic Diseases,
102

California Supreme Court, 143–44
California Tumor Registry, 91
Cancer, xv, 54, 57–58
  animal research on, 74–77
  breast, *see* Breast cancer
  DES and, 85, 143–44
  endometrial, *see* Endometrial cancer
  epidemiology of, 61–64
  ovarian, 83, 96–97, 129–30, 179
*Cancer* (journal), 128
Cancer Research Campaign, 186
Cancer and Steroid Hormones Study (CASH), 114–17, 119–25, 146
Carcinoma-in-situ, 86, 87
Case/control studies, 64, 65
Castration, 4
  female, 6–7
Centers for Disease Control (CDC), 61, 114, 115, 128, 133, 144, 155, 157
  Family Planning Evaluation Division, 114
Chang, Min-Chueh, 22, 24, 26–27, 29–31
Chemotherapy, 58, 104–5, 147–48
Chromosomes, 9, 176
CIBA Consumer Pharmaceuticals, 162, 175
Clement XIV, Pope, 4
Cohen, Michael, 178–79
Cohn, Victor, 141
Cohort studies, 64–65
Colditz, Graham, 72, 123, 129, 154–56
Cole, Philip, 77, 80, 138, 141
Collaborative Study of Steroid Contraceptives, 127–28
Confounding factors, 65–68
Congress, U.S., 17
Conjugated estrogens, 36, 152, 153, 162
Connecticut Tumor Registry, 62

Connell, Elizabeth, 42, 82
*Contraception* (journal), 96
Contraceptives, oral, *see* Birth control pills
Corfman, Philip, 71
Coronary artery disease, 10
Coronary Drug Project Research Group, 11
Corpus luteum, 10
Crile, George, 104, 147, 148
Crosson, William, 39
Currier, Andrew, 6
Cyrus, 4
Cystic mastitis, 102

Davis, Bette, 146–47
Death Registration Area, 62
Debevoise, Thomas, 41
Depo-Provera, 180*n*
Deutsch, Helene, 13
DeVita, Vincent, 148
Diethylstilbestrol (DES), 16–19, 50, 74*n*, 77, 78, 89, 106
  animal studies of, 75
  cancer and, 85, 143–44
Diosgenin, 25
Dissection, 4–5
Djerassi, Carl, 25–26, 74*n*, 75, 84, 86
Dodds, Charles, 16
Doisy, Edward A., 8, 74
Double-blind studies, 65–66

Eli Lilly, 143, 144
Embolism, 37–39, 51
Emory University, 157
Endometrial cancer, 50, 90–98, 101, 129–30, 137, 142, 152, 164, 179
Enovid, 33, 35, 38, 40, 41, 50–52, 76
Epidemiology, 61–68
Estraderm, 162, 175
Estradiol, 9, 152, 153
Estriol, 9, 108

Estrogen, 9–12
  animal studies of, 74–77
  blood clots and, 53
  discovery of, 8, 173
  endogenous exposure to,
    168–69
  for infertility, 23
  injectable, 15–16
  and medical establishment,
    42
  during pregnancy, 18–19
  retrospective studies of, 71–73
  side effects of, 16–19
  stimulation of existing cancers
    by, 80, 83, 86, 107, 125,
    174
  warning labels on products
    containing, 174–75
  See also Birth control pills; Es-
    trogen replacement therapy
Estrogen replacement therapy
    (ERT), 15–17, 19, 35–37,
    45–47, 53, 78, 80, 114
  breast cancer and, 86, 90, 127,
    137–46, 151–59, 164, 167–
    69, 174, 181, 187
  cancer and, 54
  duration of, 76
  endometrial cancer and, 91,
    93–98
  health benefits of, 159–66,
    180–81
  market for, 43
  popularity of, 89
  publicizing, 48–50
  safe alternatives to, 181–82
  side effects of, 73
  tightening of rules for pre-
    scribing, 178
Estrone, 8, 9, 75, 108
Ether, 5
Ethinyl estradiol, 16, 17

Family Planning Association of
    Puerto Rico, 30, 39
Family Planning Perspectives, 129

Fasal, Elfriede, 102, 104, 106–8,
    122, 124, 137, 142
Federal Food, Drug and Cos-
    metic Act (1938), 28
Feminine Forever (Wilson), 48, 49,
    51, 75, 91, 137, 156, 158,
    167
Fetal development, 3, 9
Fibrocystic breast disease, 95,
    155
Finkle, William D., 94
Fisher, Bernard, 148, 184
Food and Drug Administration
    (FDA), 28, 33, 35, 36, 38,
    40–42, 45, 50–54, 71, 76, 81,
    84, 89, 95, 97, 106, 114, 162,
    174–75, 177, 178, 180n
  Advisory Committee on Ob-
    stetrics and Gynecology, 52,
    53, 92n
Ford, Betty, xvi, 104–6, 148
Framingham study, 163
Free Hospital for Women, 18,
    22, 23
Fugh-Berman, Adriane, 183,
    185n
Fulbright, Elizabeth, 105

Galen, 4, 103
Gallup organization, 82
General Motors Cancer Research
    Foundation, 168
Genetic defects, 176–77
Germ theory, 6
Glass, Andrew G., 127
Goldman, Lee, 164
Gonadotropin releasing hor-
    mone (GnRH), 179–80
Gotto, Antonio, 164–65
Grady, Hugh C., 75
Grant, Robert, 52
Gray, Laman D., Sr., 138–39,
    141, 142
Greeks, ancient, 4, 6
Greenblatt, Robert B., 49
Gusberg, Saul, 91

Guttmacher, Alan, Institute, 42, 128–29, 131, 133

Halsted, William Stewart, 104, 147
Harlap, Susan, 177
*Harrison's Principles of Internal Medicine,* 97
Harvard University Medical School, 85, 124, 138
School of Public Health, 124, 168
Health and Human Services, U.S. Department of, 63
Heart disease, 10–11
ERT and, 153, 159, 162–66, 181
tamoxifen and, 184
Heath, Clark W., Jr., 156
Hemoglobin count, 166
Henderson, I. Craig, 154, 155
Hertz, Roy, 26, 75–77, 79–82, 86, 89
Hip fractures, 160
Hippocrates, 103, 178
Holleb, Arthur, 147
Hoover, Robert, 107, 123–24, 127, 137–39, 141, 142, 145, 151–54, 157, 187
Hormone replacement therapy (HRT), 46–49, 178
breast cancer and, 151–54, 159
Hormones, 7–8
male, 9, 11
*See also* Estrogen; Progesterone
Hysterectomy, 140, 145

Ibuprofen, 26n
Imperial Cancer Research Fund, 121, 186
Infection control, 6
Infertility, 23–24, 27
Inflammatory breast cancer, 58
Inhoffen, Hans H., 16

Ireland, Jill, 147, 148
Iron, 165–66

Japanese Health and Welfare Ministry, 38n
Johns Hopkins Medical Institutions, 86, 163, 164
*Journal of the American Medical Association,* 73
*Journal of Cancer Research,* 74
*Journal of the National Cancer Institute,* 106
*Journal of Reproductive Medicine,* 95

Kaiser-Permanente Medical Centers, 93–95, 127
Kaposi's sarcoma, 61
Kaufman, David W., 96
Kelsey, Frances, 83
Knauer, Emil, 7
Kushner, Rose, 104–6, 147

Laboratorios Hormona, 25
Lacassagne, A., 75
*Lancet,* 7, 110, 184
Larrick, George F., 39, 41
Lasagna, Louis, 52
Lathrop, A. F. C., 74
Lehmann, Federico, 25
Lewison, Edward F., 75–76, 86–87, 89, 90, 103, 176
Lister, Joseph, 6
Loeb, L., 74
*Look* magazine, 49
L-phenylalanine mustard (L-Pam), 105
Lumpectomy, 147–48
Lund (Sweden) University Hospital, 122

McCormick, Katherine, 22
MacMahon, Brian, 77, 80, 138, 141

Makowski, Edgar L., 91–93
Mammography, 58, 66, 103, 105, 147, 148
Marker, Russell E., 25
Massachusetts General Hospital, 5
Mastectomy, 103–5, 146–48
Mead-Johnson, 92n, 137
*Medical Letter, The,* 49
Meier, Diane, 162
Melatonin, 179
Memorial Sloan-Kettering Cancer Center, 41n, 147
Menopause, 7, 11, 12
  avoidance of, 46–47
  breast cancer after, 72
  as disease, 13–16, 45
  estrogen levels at, 8
  estrogen replacement for, *see* Estrogen replacement therapy
  ovariectomy as cure for, 6
Menstrual cycle
  age at first, 168, 169
  estrogen levels during, 8–10, 15–16, 152–53
*Merck Manual, The,* 14–15, 168, 174
*Merck Index, The,* 18
Mestranol, 31, 32
Metastasis, 58, 80, 103, 125, 126
Miami, University of, School of Medicine, 185
Miscarriage, 18
Morton, William, 5, 74, 104
Moskowitz, Myron, 59
Murphy, Gerald, 126–27

Nachtigall, Lila, 160
National Cancer Institute (NCI), 42, 62–65, 75, 79, 81, 93, 105, 107, 114, 123, 127, 137, 138, 145, 148, 183, 184
National Center for Health Statistics, 63, 64, 68
National Conferences on Breast Cancer, 59, 77, 80, 85, 90, 138, 147
National Council of Churches, 31n
National Health and Nutrition Survey, 163, 164
National Heart, Lung and Blood Institute, 11
National Heart Association, 163
National Institute on Aging, 142
National Institute of Child Health and Human Development (NICHD), 26, 114, 115, 116
  Center for Population Research, 114
National Institutes of Health (NIH), 11, 26, 75, 79, 102, 163, 180
  Consensus Development Conference, 161
  Office of Research on Women's Health, 177
National Women's Health Network, 83, 175
  Midlife Women's Health Issues section, 161
Nelson, Gaylord, 81–83, 114
New Drug Application (NDA), 28
*New England Journal of Medicine,* 85, 93, 94, 96, 139, 144, 152, 153, 164
*Newsweek,* 59n, 156
New York Academy of Sciences, 79
New York State Court of Appeals, 144
*New York Times, The,* 85, 126, 148
New York University Medical Center, 160
New Zealand National Case-Control Study, 151
Nicaea, Council of, 4
Nolvadex, *see* Tamoxifen
Norethandrolone, 27
Norethindrone, 25–29, 31

Norethynodrel, 26–29, 31–33
Norinyl, 26*n*
Norplant, 32*n*, 180*n*
Norquen, 92
Nurses Health Study, 124–25,
    127, 154, 155, 163–64, 174


Oracon, 92
Oral contraceptives, *see* Birth
    control pills
Ortho-Novum SQ, 92
Ortho-Novum 7/7/7, 97, 175
Ortho Pharmaceutical Corpora-
    tion, 42, 92*n*, 97, 131, 175
Ory, Howard W., 116
Osler, William, 173
Osteoporosis, 159–62, 178, 181,
    182
Ovariectomy, 139–40, 145, 161
    for breast cancer, 7, 72, 74,
        77, 126, 187
    for menopause, 6
Ovaries, 3–7
    cancer of, 83, 96–97, 129–30,
        179
    deficiency of, menopause seen
        as, 14
    hormones of, 7–8; *see also* Es-
        trogen
Ovulation, 10, 152–53
    inhibition of, 23–24; *see also*
        Birth control pills
Ovulen, 52
Oxford University, 121


Paffenbarger, Ralph, 101–2, 104,
    106–8, 110, 114, 122, 124,
    137, 142
Paget's disease, 58
Paniagua, Miguel E., 39
Parke-Davis, 25
Pascuzzi, Chris A., 51–52
Pasteur, Louis, 5–6
Patterson, James T., 103
Pearson, Cindy, 175–76, 181–82

Pelvic inflammatory disease,
    129
Pennsylvania State University, 22,
    24, 32*n*
Persians, ancient, 4
Peto, Richard, 185*n*
Pfeffer, Robert, 144–45
Phoenicians, 4
Pike, Malcolm, 108–10, 114, 115,
    117, 119, 121, 131, 138, 154,
    168, 179, 187
Pill, the, *see* Birth control pills
Pincus, Gregory Goodman, 22,
    24, 26–31, 37
Pineal gland, 179
Pituitary gland, 10
Placenta, estrogen production
    by, 9
Planned Parenthood, 21, 27, 30,
    35, 38, 40, 42, 120, 129,
    180*n*
Poliomyelitis, 102
Population Council, 41, 180*n*,
    182
Pregnancy
    breast cancer during, 72
    breast cancer risk and, 108–
        10, 115–17, 168–69, 176
    DES and, 18–19, 75, 89
    estrogen levels during, 8
    natural hazards of, 177
Premarin, 95
*Preventing Pregnancy, Protecting
    Health* (Guttmacher Insti-
    tute), 128–30, 133
Primate research, 76–77
Primilut N, 35
Progesterone, 10, 15–16
    for infertility, 23–24
    isolation of, 11
    synthesis of, 25–26
    *See also* Birth control pills;
        Hormone replacement ther-
        apy
Puberty, 10
Public Citizen Health Research
    Group, xvii

Public Health Services, U.S.,
  Cancer Control Program, 77

Radiation therapy, 58, 148
Ramazzini, Bernardino, 168,
  169, 186
Reagan, Nancy, 148–49
Rees, Dai A., 186
Relative risk, 93–94
Reproductive Study Center, 22, 23
Rexall Drug, 143
Rock, John, 22–24, 27, 30, 35, 37
Rockefeller, John D., Jr., 41
Rockefeller, Margaretta
  "Happy," xvi, 41n, 105, 106
Rockefeller, Nelson, 41n, 105
Rockefeller Foundation, 42
Rockefeller Institute, 41
*Roe* v. *Wade* (1973), 31
Rollin, Betty, 105
Roman Catholic Church, 4, 5, 30
Rosemond, George P., 147
Ross, Ronald K., 144–45
RU-486, 28n
Rutqvist, Lars E., 185

Salonen, Jukka T., 165
Sanger, Margaret, 21–22, 28
Sartwell, Philip E., 53, 85–86
Scandinavian National Case-
  Control Study, 151
Schairer, Catherine, 151
Schering, 16
Schlesselman, James J., 117, 119,
  121, 123
Schmidt, Alexander, 95
Seaman, Barbara, 33n, 39, 75
Searle, G. D., corporation, 26,
  27, 31, 33, 35, 38–40, 42,
  50–53, 81, 95, 167
Searle, John G., 40
Semmelweis, Ludwig Ignaz Phil-
  ipp, 6
Senate, U.S., 79, 81
  Subcommittee on Health, 137

Sequential birth control pills, 92
Sexually-transmitted diseases
  (STDs), 129, 182
Shimkin, Michael B., 75
Silverberg, Steven, 91–93
Smith, Donald C., 94
Smith, George, 18–19, 75
Smith, Olive, 18–19, 75
Somlo, Emeric, 25
Southern California, University
  of, School of Medicine, 108,
  110
Southern Presbyterian church,
  31n
Spontaneous abortion, 18
Squibb, E. R., Pharmaceuticals,
  143
Stadel, Bruce V., 116–17, 119,
  121, 123
Stampfer, Mier J., 163–64
Stem cells, 57
Stern, Rigoni, 168–69
Strax, Philip, 103
Stroke, 163
Supreme Court, U.S., 30–31, 144
Surgery
  antiseptic, 6
  for breast cancer, 103–5, 146–48
  and development of anesthe-
    sia, 5
Surveillance, Epidemilogy and
  End Results (SEER) pro-
  gram, 62–65, 114, 123
Syntex Laboratories, 25–27, 31,
  42, 92n

Tamoxifen, 182–86
Terry, Luther, 174
Testicles, 3
  effect of progestins on, 30
  estrogen production by, 9
Testosterone, 9, 126
  isolation of, 11
  for menopausal women, 17
Thalidomide, 83
Thau, Rosemary, 180n

Thrombophlebitis, 39, 41
Thyroid hormones, 7
Tri-Norinyl, 26n
Tyrer, Louise, 120

U.K. National Case-Control
    Study Group, 121, 131, 144,
    151, 157
U.K. Committee on the Safety of
    Medicines, 53, 184
U.S. Census, 62, 68
Upjohn Pharmaceuticals, 143
Urban Jermone A., 147
Uterus, 4, 5
    cancer of, *see* Endometrial can-
    cer
    changes in, during menstrual
    cycle, 10

Vaginal cancer, 85, 143–44
Vaughn, Paul, 29–30, 40

Vesalius, Andreas, 5
Vessey, Martin, 85–86
*Vogue* magazine, 48

Warren, John, 5
Washington, University of, 93,
    94
*Washington Memo,* 129
Wilson, Robert A., 45–50, 73, 75,
    76, 137, 156, 158, 167
Wingo, Phyllis, 116, 120–21,
    146
Wolfe, Sidney, xvii, 36
Worcester Foundation for Exper-
    imental Biology, 22
World Health Organization
    (WHO), 84, 127–28, 180n
Wyeth-Ayerst, 32n

Ziel, Harry K., 94
Zondek, Bernhardt, 8